TURN ON THE TAP . . .
AND REAP THE BENEFITS OF ONE OF THE GREATEST HEALTH DISCOVERIES OF ALL TIME!

Learn the crucial role water plays in these and many other conditions and ailments:

HEART DISEASE AND STROKE—water is essential to help prevent clogging of arteries in the heart and brain

INFECTION—water may increase the efficiency of the immune system to combat infections and cancer cells

DEPRESSION—water helps the body naturally replenish its supply of the neurotransmitter serotonin

SLEEP DISORDERS—water is needed for the production of nature's sleep regulator, melatonin

LACK OF ENERGY—water generates electrical and magnetic energy in every body cell, providing a natural power boost

ADDICTION—water can help eliminate addictive urges for caffeine, alcohol, and some drugs

OSTEOPOROSIS—water is an aid to strong bone formation

LEUKEMIA AND LYMPHOMA—water normalizes the blood-manufacturing systems that can aid in the prevention of many forms of cancer

ATTENTION DEFICIT—a well-hydrated brain is continually energized to imprint new information in its memory banks.

WATER: FOR HEALTH, FOR HEALING, FOR LIFE

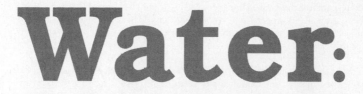

Water:

for Health, for Healing, for Life

YOU'RE NOT SICK, YOU'RE THIRSTY!

F. Batmanghelidj, M.D.

WARNER BOOKS

NEW YORK   BOSTON

This book is not intended as a substitute for medical advice of physicians. The reader should regularly consult a physician in all matters relating to his or her health, and particularly in respect of any symptoms that may require diagnosis or medical attention.

Some of the material in this book originally appeared in *Your Body's Many Cries for Water*, which was first published in 1992 and updated in 1995.

Copyright © 2003 Fereydoon Batmanghelidj, M.D.
All rights reserved.

Warner Books

Time Warner Book Group
1271 Avenue of the Americas, New York, NY 10020
Visit our Web site at www.twbookmark.com

Printed in the United States of America

First Printing: June 2003
10 9 8 7 6 5 4 3

Library of Congress-in-Publication Data

Batmanghelidj, F.
    Water, for health, for healing, for life : you're not sick, you're thirsty! /
F. Batmanghelidj.
        p. cm.
    Includes index.
    ISBN 0-446-69074-0
        1. Hydrotherapy. 2. Water—Health aspects. 3. Dehydration (Physiology)
I. Title.

RM252 .B367 2003
615.8'53—dc21

                                                                    2002191013

Cover design by Brigid Pearson
Cover photo by Patrick J. LaCroix/Getty Images
Book design and text composition by L & G McRee

To Our Creator with Awe, Humility, Dedication, and Love

Also, dedicated to all who suffered because of our past limitations in medical knowledge.

"The worse sin toward our fellow creatures is not to hate them, but to be indifferent to them; that's the essence of inhumanity."

George Bernard Shaw, 1897

Altruism and selfishness are both characteristics and mechanisms of self-protection. Selfish traits compel us to self-indulge at the expense of others. When a society is made mostly of such people, a vicious circle of chaos will develop. Altruism, on the other hand, is the quality and product of unselfishness, prompting endeavors that benefit society and humankind, the survival and progress of which also serve the altruist.

This book is designed to serve society and all decent people in it who contribute to its integrity, advancement, health, wealth, and prosperity.

ACKNOWLEDGMENT

To medical maverick Professor Emeritus Howard Spiro, M.D., of Yale University. He was the first medical scientist to realize the merit of my clinical research and introduce it to Western medicine; he published my editorial article, "A New and Natural Method of Treatment of Peptic Ulcer Disease," in his *Journal of Clinical Gastroenterology* in June 1983. His interest and encouragement gave me incentive to pursue my research to this date, the product of which is the information you have in your hands.

AUTHOR'S NOTE

The information and recommendations on water intake presented in this book are based on training, personal experience, very extensive research, and other publications of the author on the topic of water metabolism of the body. The author of this book does not dispense medical advice or prescribe the use or the discontinuance of any medications as a form of treatment without the advice of an attending physician, either directly or indirectly. The intent of the author, based on the most recent knowledge of microanatomy and molecular physiology, is only to offer information on the importance of water to well-being, and to help inform the public of the damaging effects of chronic dehydration to the body—from childhood to old age. This book is not intended as a replacement for sound medical advice from a physician. On the contrary, sharing of the information contained in this book with the attending physician is highly desirable. Application of the information and recommendations described herein are undertaken at the individual's own risk. The adoption of the information should be in strict compliance with the instructions given herein. No reader, and especially those with past history of major diseases and under professional supervision, or those with severe renal disease, should make use of the information contained herein without the supervision of their attending physician.

CONTENTS

PREFACE

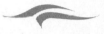

THE DAWN OF A NEW MEDICAL ERA

Only if you begin to suffer from a health problem that may eventually kill you will you begin to search high and low for an explanation and solution to your predicament. Until then, you cannot appreciate what an emotionally draining impact a doctor's visit and the pronouncement of his or her serious findings has on the life and soul of another person. Let us hope you or anyone you care for never confronts such a situation— which thousands face daily. The reason we have a health-care crisis in America today is because many diseases prematurely devastate and kill millions of people. At the same time, the health-care crisis costs us about $1.2 trillion in 2001, and it is predicted that this cost will increase by 11 percent every year.

It is true that we are scientifically the most advanced nation in the world and spend billions of dollars a year on medical research. If you look at any recently published medical textbooks, however, you will see page upon page of explanation about diseases that kill; yet when the authors of these books reach the point of having to shed light on the cause of the disease, they confess—"etiology unknown." This means most doctors do not know the cause of the major diseases of the human body, yet society has given them license to prescribe various treatments that often do not benefit their patients, but can slowly and prematurely kill them. The good news is that this license is about to be withdrawn.

What you are about to read is new knowledge, and represents a new perspective within the science of physiology—not a form of science used by drug manufacturers, but the discipline of science that defines the way living tissues and organs within the body work *naturally*. This book deals with some important health problems and the cause and natural correction—cure—of these problems. When the cause and cure of any health problem becomes clear, the use of excessive language and tongue-twisting jargon becomes unnecessary. What you will read here is based on extensive clinical and scientific research. I have researched, studied, and written about the information in this book for more than twenty-two years, in addition to my medical training, which began in 1950, when I entered St. Mary's Hospital Medical School of London University.

The topic I am about to discuss is the physiological ramifications and metabolic complications of chronic unintentional dehydration as the primary cause of many serious diseases. Some say it is the greatest breakthrough in modern medicine.

This simple presentation about some of our modern health problems is an introduction to the eventual science- and logic-based transformation of medicine all over the world. It is prepared with the immediate "shot-in-the-arm" needs of society in mind, particularly for the fifteen million asthmatic children whose parents urgently need to understand the cause of this disease and its simple, cost-free prevention and potentially lifesaving treatment.

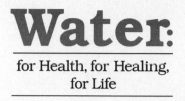

Water:

for Health, for Healing, for Life

CHAPTER 1

WHERE DID MODERN MEDICINE GO WRONG?

The greatest tragedy in medical history in my opinion is the assumption that dry mouth is the only sign of the body's water needs. Based on this mistaken assumption, modern medicine has made three other confounding mistakes that have cost society dearly. Let us look at these four mistaken assumptions.

1. The whole structure of modern medicine is built on the pitifully flawed premise that *dry mouth is the only sign of dehydration*. This false premise is responsible for the lack of understanding about various painful health problems that result in premature death to many millions of people. They suffer because they do not know they are seriously thirsty. Modern "science-based" medicine is structured upon the simple dry mouth mistake that became established many years ago. In 1764, Albrecht von Haller, a German, first claimed dry mouth as a sign of thirst. In 1918, Walter Bradford Cannon, an English doctor, supported Haller's views; since he was an influential person, his views became fashionable

and are reflected in accepted scientific literature to this day. Frenchman Moritz Schiff, however, had claimed in 1867 that thirst is a general sensation: "It is no more a local sensation than hunger." We now know that Haller and Cannon were wrong— but since theirs were the views that took root in the infrastructure of medicine, the same mistake has been passed on from one generation of medical students to another until the present day. This traditional flaw in the scientific understanding of the human body's water regulation altered the path of medicine. Schiff understood the human body better.

Actually, dry mouth is not a sign to rely on. The human body uses a different logic: To be able to chew and swallow food, and to facilitate and lubricate this function, ample saliva is produced, even if the rest of the body is short of water. In any case, water is too important to the body to signal its shortage only through the experience of a dry mouth. The human body has many other sophisticated signals to indicate when it is short of water. The body can suffer from deep dehydration without showing a dry mouth. Dehydration produces severe symptoms, even to the point of causing life-threatening crises. Modern medicine has confused these symptoms of internal, localized droughts and has identified them as different diseases. As a result, toxic medications are prescribed to treat "diseases" rather than the dehydration.

Dry mouth is one of the very last indicators of dehydration of the body. By the time dry mouth becomes an indicator of water shortage, many delicate functions of the body have been shut down and prepared for deletion. This is exactly how the aging process is established—through a loss of enzyme functions. A dehydrated body loses sophistication and versatility. One example is juvenile diabetes, in which the insulin-producing cells of the pancreas are sacrificed as a result of persistent dehydration.

2. The second major mistake in the basic science of medicine is the thinking that *water is a simple substance that only dissolves and circulates different things*. Water is not a simple inert substance. It has two primary properties in the body. The first one is its life-sustaining properties. The other, more important, role of water is its life-giving functions. Modern medicine recognizes only the life-sustaining properties of water. That is why chronic unintentional dehydration is ultimately an unrecognized life-threatening process. You need to recognize and understand the process to save your health and your life—naturally.

3. The third serious error in medicine is the premise that *the human body can regulate efficiently its water intake throughout the life span of the person*. As we grow older, we lose our perception of thirst and fail to drink adequately, until the plumlike cells in vital organs become prunelike and can no longer sustain life. We need to recognize the onset of dehydration and its manifestations to prevent the irreversible stages of the process.

4. The fourth nail in the coffin of present-day medicine is the thought that *any fluid can replace the*

water needs of the body. This is a major problem at present. Some of the manufactured beverages in common use do not function in the body like natural water. If you begin to understand the natural reason some plants manufacture caffeine, or even cocaine, you will then recognize the problem.

The information in this book is about one of the greatest of all health discoveries in the world, because it exposes an important tragedy in medical history— the erroneous assumption that the dry mouth state is the only sign of the body's water needs. Simply put, *the new scientific understanding is that chronic unintentional dehydration in the human body can manifest itself in as many ways as we in medicine have invented diseases.* We have created an opportunity for the drug industry to thrive, and have given birth to the current "sick-care" health system, at the expense of people's precious lives and resources. The sick-care system survives and thrives when people are continuously sick. This is exactly what is going on now.

Tragically, the medical breakthrough about dehydration as the origin of most health problems is not reaching the public through the commerce-directed health-maintenance systems in this country. If it did, it would mean the rapid extinction of these systems. Yet there is no sane reason why tens of millions in our society should be medicated when all they suffer from is dehydration.

The statements in this introductory chapter are not meant to reflect badly on the dedicated staff employed within the sick-care system, who daily render compassionate service to the unfortunate sick. They are not to be blamed for the fundamental mistakes in standard treatment protocols in medicine. The blame is directed at the medical professionals in powerful positions and the national health institutes that have the power to correct the problem, but have shown reluctance to do so.

Mainstream medicine and its fund-raising sidekicks will not of their own accord abandon pharmaceutical medicine. Why? They do not want to allow *natural* solutions to the health problems of society to get clearance and reach the public. This book is designed to upset this self-serving trend, which benefits only the commercial health-care systems in our advanced society, to the detriment of the people.

It is now crystal clear that the human body has many different ways of showing its general or local water needs. These manifestations of drought in the body have been assumed to be indicators of this or that disease condition. Based on this ignorance, and protected and coddled by the pharmaceutical industry, mainstream medicine has labeled the different complications of dehydration as various "diseases." On the basis of this erroneous assumption, the trusting American public has to pay ever-increasing health-care costs with their health and hard-earned money.

We must understand that persistent dehydration brings about a continuously changing new chemical state in the body. When a new dehydration-produced chemical state becomes fully established, it causes many structural changes, even to the genetic blueprints of the body. This is why prevention of dehydration is crucial. This is also why childhood asthma is a major health issue with me, as is noninfectious earache in infants. Dehydration, to the point of causing asthma in children, can ultimately cause genetic damage, autoimmune diseases, and even cancer in their later years.

Understanding chronic dehydration will clear the way for the development of an infinitely more people-friendly health-care system. It will be possible in my estimation to have a decidedly healthier and productive nation at 30 percent of the present health-care costs. As you see, I am not promoting a moneymaking product. I am only sharing a unique medical insight and the outcome of my many years of research that will help medical professionals and the public understand the basic cause of so many conditions of ill health.

We are in the twenty-first century, yet even at this stage of our development, the outward manifestations of regional dehydration have not been understood by us in medicine. We have always looked for a drug solution to throw at a health concern. We have not succeeded at limiting these health concerns; rather, we have constantly expanded the list and thrown more drugs at them. We have truly caused a costly chaos in the name of modern medicine, with no end in sight. We now have significant problems that beg urgent solutions. As Albert Einstein observed: "The significant problems we have cannot be solved at the same level of thinking with which we created them." We obviously need a new approach to medical science to solve our health problems.

The solution to the present human-made and drug-industry-protected health problems of society can only be physiology-based. Understanding the molecular physiology of dehydration will restructure the future practice of clinical medicine. It will cause a *fundamental paradigm change* in the science of medicine. By showing the way to enhance the natural healing powers of the body within the discipline of physiology, the pharmaceutical approach to our present health problems will be completely replaced. The primary focus in medicine will become *disease prevention* rather than its protracted, cost-intensive, and invasive treatment protocols.

THE NEW LEVEL OF THINKING IN MEDICINE

What is a paradigm, and how can it be changed in clinical medicine? A paradigm is the basic infrastructural information, assumption, or understanding on which knowledge within a discipline of thought develops. As an example, based on the fundamental understanding that planet Earth is a sphere, all geographic maps and models reflect the roundness of Earth. This understanding is the basic paradigm to the design of all geographic maps. The dramatic changes produced by the realization that Earth is not flat, as originally perceived, revolutionized the knowledge we now possess about the structure of the universe. When a paradigm leads a discipline of thought toward a dead end (as in the case of a flat Earth), for those who can stand back and impartially reassess the infrastructure of knowledge, often a new paradigm emerges. All it takes is a thought-triggering association or observation.

When a valid paradigm that is basic to a major discipline of thought emerges, it illuminates the path to a vast new domain of knowledge, like a flash of lightning that reveals all in the darkness of night. A new paradigm removes restrictions and barriers and makes future progress within a discipline of thought possible.

A new paradigm is more easily born when there is a specific need and a purpose to find a solution. A solution does not establish significance unless a definite need to the emerging solution is also recognized. The following story may help explain this thought.

Sir Alexander Fleming was the Nobel laureate recognized to have discovered penicillin. He was a Scottish scientist who worked at the Wright-Fleming Institute of St. Mary's Hospital Medical School of London University when I was a medical student there in the 1950s. Many medical students have an emotional urge to become discoverers. I was no exception. Since childhood, I had been driven to study medicine and become someone who could positively affect the lives of people who fell sick.

In the introductory bacteriology course, students were divided into small groups and assigned to different tutors. Luck placed me in the tutorial group assigned to Sir Alexander. He was a refined and humble man. At the end of the tutorial, I gathered enough courage to ask him a question, the answer to which has deeply influenced me ever since.

I asked him, "Sir Alexander, is there a special way to become a discoverer in medicine?" He looked at me and pondered my naive question. After a pause, in a very refined Scottish brogue he replied, "Need and purpose." He explained that with the increasing introduction of different surgical treatment procedures into medical practice, there was an ever-increasing rate of fatal bacterial complications. To find an agent that would stop bacterial infections in the human body became a most urgent need that established a purpose and resolve for those in bacterial research. "Need" was the mother of penicillin's discovery, and "purpose" the impetus of its development for human application.

THE BIRTH OF A NEW SCIENTIFIC TRUTH IN MEDICINE

History tells us that every so often, through basic discoveries of the applied techniques of nature, important leaps of progress have become possible. Humankind, because of these fortuitous happenstances and flashes of insight, has unraveled many of the secrets employed in its creation.

One such happenstance seems to have revealed itself in 1979. I had become a political prisoner of Islamic revolutionaries and was being held in the Iranian prison of Evin. While facing the possibility of execution, I discovered one late night that two glasses of water could relieve even the severest abdominal pain associated with peptic ulcer disease.

A prisoner needed medication for his excruciating ulcer pain which had him doubled up and unable to walk by himself. Two friends were supporting him. The guards had not responded to his repeated pleas to be taken to the prison hospital. It was after eleven at night when he was brought to me. I was a prisoner myself and had no medication to give the man, who was truly in agony. I explained to him that I had no medicine to give him. His face showed even more pain than before. Instead of medication, I gave him two glasses of water. Within minutes, his ulcer pain became less severe. In eight minutes, it disappeared completely. This confirmed for me the abdominal-pain-relieving effect of water in a "disease" condition (I had relieved my own abdominal pain with water during a period of solitary confinement when I refused food for several days). I encouraged one after another of the inmates who had this same classic pain to take water in place of medications that were sometimes available.

During the ensuing two and a half years of my imprisonment, I successfully treated well over three thousand stress-induced peptic ulcer disease cases with tap water only. It became obvious to me that these people were really and only thirsty. They were presenting their dehydration in the form of a painful crisis situation that we in the medical profession had labeled a "disease" condition. As a last defense at my trial—about fifteen months into my imprisonment—I presented a scientific article to be released for publication. I told the judge that even if he had me shot, to please not lose the information. "It is the greatest medical discovery in history," I said. By then I had already treated a few hundred fellow prisoners in the confined prison block where I was housed.

The judge later came to me and said: "You have made a tremendous discovery; I wish you luck in the future." That was the first indication that I had a future and could continue my work.

As acknowledgment of my discovery, I was not executed but given a three-year sentence. My life was spared because of what I had discovered in the prison. All my personal assets, however, were confiscated. After twenty-three months, the prison warden told me the authorities had discovered I was "not the bad person they had been led to believe," and they were considering an early release for me. I thanked him, but said I wanted to stay on in prison a while longer. I was in the middle of clinical observations on the effect of water as a treatment of various stress-induced health problems, including bleeding peptic ulcer conditions. I explained to him that as a sort of stress laboratory, Evin was unique. Needless to say, the warden was surprised. He thought he was doing me a great favor by wanting to release me before the end of my sentence. He agreed that my work was important, however, and that I should be given the opportunity to complete what I was doing. I had for some time believed that my coming to prison had not been a chance event. I was destined to make my discovery that the human body has sophisticated crisis calls for water when it is stressed and becomes dehydrated. I stayed in prison an additional four months and reached certain clinical conclusions that now needed scientific explanations. After two years and seven months of imprisonment, I was released with an official acclaim for my discovery.

During my prison time, I gained much new understanding about the physiological effects of water and its relationship to many disease conditions. It all started with abdominal pain. I published the first announcement of my discovery in the *Iranian Medical Association Journal* while I was still in prison. A translation of the article was sent to America and was eventually restructured for publication as a guest editorial in the *Journal of Clinical Gastroenterology* in June 1983.

THE STEPS IN SHAPING PRESENT-DAY MEDICINE

The explanations that follow are based on clinical observations made in one of the worst stress laboratories in the world. These observations have given birth to a new physiology-based explanation of how diseases of the body occur. My findings have been presented at several international gatherings of scientists. Detailed scientific explanations that support my findings have also been published.

It does not require a detailed knowledge of science to understand that water should be used to prevent and cure certain dehydration-produced disease conditions. Nor does the use of water as a "medicine" require Food and Drug Administration (FDA) approval. Water is the main source of life, and everyone knows about it. Still, there is shameful ignorance about the health dangers we expose our bodies to when we do not drink enough water. Our saving grace is that the human body understands the role of water in maintaining its physiological and physical well-being, even though mainstream medicine does not. It seems we doctors have not been well informed about the different functional relationships of water in the human body. We have been caught in a most embarrassing situation. We do not yet know when the human body is truly thirsty. We do not understand what happens if the body does not receive adequate water on a regular basis.

The current practice of clinical medicine is based on the application of pharmacological chemistry to the human body. At medical schools, more than six hundred teaching hours are allocated to the use of pharmaceutical products. Only a few hours are allocated to instructions on diet and food. It seems that in most "disease" conditions, medical educators are trying to force the test-tube understanding of chemistry into the human body.

The trouble is, pharmaceutical or chemical products do not cure most disease conditions. Nor are most of these products safe for long-term use. They only temporarily mask and silence the outward manifestations of the problem. No matter how seemingly scientific, sophisticated, and appealing the justifications for the use of these chemical products might seem, they often do not remove the medical problem—except for the use of antibiotics in infections. People with hypertension, who begin treatment with diuretics or other chemicals, are not cured. They are told they must continue the treatment for the rest of their lives. They often need to supplement the diuretic and use other types of medication at the same time. People with rheumatoid arthritis are not permanently cured by any of the many analgesics on the market. They have to use analgesic medications for the rest of their pain-filled lives. No diabetic is cured; no person with myasthenia gravis is cured; no person with muscular dystrophy is cured. How is it possible that, despite extensive research, no cure for any one of the prevalent conditions such as heartburn, dyspepsia, back pain, rheumatoid arthritis, migraine, or asthma has been found?

Dehydration eventually causes loss of some functions and produces damage (pathology). The various signals or symptoms produced during severe and lasting dehydration have been interpreted by doctors as various disease conditions of unknown origin. The signal, however, is actually for water shortage, and the local damage is because of water shortage. Because doctors don't recognize chronic dehydration as the original cause, the "disease" conditions receive all sorts of explanations and labels, and all of them are said to have an unknown cause. This is the basic mistake that has distorted the truth in medicine and devastated people needing professional advice and guidance for their health issues. This is the crack through which all past research on the origin of some disease conditions has fallen.

CHAPTER 2

Water, water everywhere, yet not enough did we drink.
Water, water everywhere, still our bodies
did shriek and shrink.

WATER—THE BIZARRE AND
THE SIMPLE

The human body is about 75 percent water and 25 percent solid matter. The brain is said to be 85 percent water and is extremely sensitive to any dehydration or depletion of its water content. The brain is bathed constantly in salty cerebrospinal fluid. The water content of the body is called the solvent, and the solid matter that is dissolved in the water is called the solute. The chemical understanding of the human body brought about an almost total concentration of research into the detailed molecular composition and minute fluctuations of the solid matter in the body. Thus a chemical-pharmaceutical perception of the human body took shape, resulting in the development of the "medical-industrial system." Adherence to the understanding that it is primarily the body's solid composition that governs all its functions has produced much misinformation and has contributed to the present chaotic status of medicine.

The flaw in the above approach to understanding the body lies in the fact that, even with all our amassed knowledge, the human body is still an almost unknown structure. We know no more than 10 percent of how the body functions and is integrated chemically.

The practice of clinical medicine today benefits the manufacturing and commercial arms of the health-care system. The ignorance-promoting and money-making solutes focus is strictly guarded and forcefully dispensed—it is good for selling drugs. Although the knowledge of the physiology of the human body is advanced, the practice of clinical medicine does not benefit from the advancement of this discipline of science.

WE ARE STILL WATER-DEPENDENT

The role of water in the bodies of all living species, humans included, has not changed since the earliest creation of life in water.

When life on land became an objective—the stressful adventure beyond known boundaries and the immediate vicinity of water supply—a gradually refined body-water-preservation system and drought-management system had to be created. In other words, the body began to adapt to transient dehydration. Over time, this drought-management process became permanent—and currently exists in the body of modern humans.

Even now, when humans are under stress or confronting situations that may be perceived as stressful, the physiological translation of that stress reflects a water-regulation process. It is as if nothing has changed from the first time water-dwelling species ventured beyond their water supply. A similar process for rationing water reserves and an anticipated limited future supply becomes the responsibility of a complex system in the body. This multisystem water-distribution process remains in operation until the body receives unmistakable signals that it has once more gained access to an adequate water supply.

One of the unavoidable processes in the body-water rationing phase is the ruthlessness with which the body functions are monitored. No structure receives more than its predetermined share of water, based on its functional importance. The brain takes absolute priority over all the other systems.

Thinking that tea, coffee, alcohol, and manufactured beverages can substitute for the pure natural water needs of the body is an elementary mistake, particularly in a body that is stressed by confronting daily problems. It is true that these beverages contain water, but most of them also contain dehydrating substances, such as caffeine. These substances rid the body of the water they are dissolved in, plus additional water from the body's reserves. When you drink coffee, tea, or even a beer, your body gets rid of more water than is contained in the drink. If you measure your urine volume after the beverage is taken, you will see that you have passed more urine than the volume of the drink. Another way the body loses water after drinking hot beverages is through perspiration from the pores of the skin to cool the body that has been warmed from the inside.

The economic principles are the same in the body as they are in society. The law of supply and demand rules absolutely. When there is a comparative shortage of a needed substance, a strict rationing system rules the marketplace of the body with an iron fist.

When the human body is dehydrated, it redistributes and regulates the amount of available water. Within the body, alarms signal to show that areas in question are in short supply, much like the light signal that goes on when a car is running low on gas or oil. The available water is rationed and used where needed. The presence of water will ultimately regulate the production mechanisms in a drought-stricken area of the body.

When chronic dehydration begins to set in, up to a certain level the shutdown of water-dependent functions is silent because there is a reserve capacity for endurance. As time passes and the body becomes more and more dehydrated, however, a threshold is reached where the system becomes inadequate for the responsibilities thrust on one or another function of the body. Depending on the type of demand, the organ or organs in the firing line of activity begin to indicate their particular signal of inadequacy.

While the various signals produced by the water distributors and drought managers indicate regional body thirst and drought, and can naturally and simply be relieved by an increased intake of water, they are, instead, often improperly and ignorantly dealt with by highly potent chemical products. Because many doctors are not educated about the symptoms of dehydration and the importance of the fluid in the body, they often diagnose the problem incorrectly. Many physicians mistake dehydration for one or another disease and treat the symptoms with medication rather than water. The result: Pharmaceutical companies get rich, patients are not cured, and doctors are helpless in dealing with often recurring disease states of the body.

Silencing the different signal systems of water shortage in the body with chemical products can be immediately detrimental to the patient's body cells, including the genetic apparatus. Chronic dehydration can have a permanently damaging impact on a person's descendants. While the human body is entirely dependent on the many complicated functions of water for its survival, it has not developed a water-storage system in the same way it stores fat. The dehydration-produced loss of body efficiency and resulting loss of chemical know-how and function in one generation can be projected onto the next generation. If the root cause of a disease state is dehydration, the same malfunctioning sensor systems that permit dehydration to establish in an individual can eventually be inherited by some of the offspring. This is why asthma, allergies, and heartburn are very serious conditions that should be prevented by full hydration at all times. It is essential to become educated about the functions of water in the body at all ages. This is how disease can be prevented in individuals and the next-generation descendants.

We must learn to recognize the symptoms of dehydration and understand that the treatment is simple: water. It's vital to our health.

In an article in the *New England Journal of Medicine*, September 20, 1984, Dr. Paddy Phillips and seven associates showed that elderly men were far less able to recognize their body thirst than younger men in the same experimental setting. When the elderly were dehydrated, they seemed not to feel thirsty. Even when blood tests showed an obvious water shortage in the body, and even when water was within reach, some of the persons tested did not seem to want to drink. They remained dehydrated. An editorial in *The Lancet* of November 3, 1984, discussed the experimental results of Phillips and his associates and mentioned other findings to support the conclusion that in the elderly, the thirst mechanism is gradually lost. Steen, Lundgren, and Isaksson reported in *The Lancet* of January 12, 1985, that, in their long-term observation, they had discovered significant body-water loss in the elderly—about 3.5 to 6 liters over ten years. This is a large loss from the fluid content of the body—mostly from inside the cells.

To give further scientific support to the new paradigm, let us briefly mention the single most important point of a scientific paper by Ephraim Katchalski-Katzir of the Weizmann Institute. The far-reaching significance of the finding is that proteins and enzymes function more efficiently in solutions of lower viscosity. They need adequate water in their

immediate environment to "diffuse" and work efficiently. In other words, in solutions of higher viscosity—produced by the loss of water from the cell
content—the enzyme system within the cell becomes
less efficient. As an analogy, could a competitive
swimmer have room to practice in a pool full of kids?
Obviously not. The same logic seems to apply to the
enzymes in the cells of the body that "swim in cell
water" to contact their chemical partners and to produce a desirable outcome.

A gradual loss of sensations in the body should be
assumed to involve all aspects of the sensory mechanisms. As we grow older, we gradually lose sharpness of
vision and become dependent on glasses. We lose
sexual appetite. Our ability to hear some ranges of
sound is gradually lost. Our feelings become less tender
and lose alertness; our emotional stimulation becomes
dull and less satisfying, and so on. These are the
apparent outward manifestations of a gradual loss of
the ability to differentiate and respond to the stimulation of the senses at some time or another in the life
of any individual.

Although we do not know how and when the
dulling of senses in the body begins, logical interpre-
tation from the above scientific experiments, in addition to my personal observations, has led me to
believe that reliance on our sense of thirst, and
waiting to feel thirsty before we drink water, is the
basic problem. The most significant and major complication of dehydration is the loss of a number of
essential amino acids that are used to manufacture
neurotransmitters.

A major hidden advantage to adequate hydration seems to be the increased efficiency of the many thousands of proteins and enzymes whose physiological responsibilities are not yet recognized. They, too, will be more efficiently integrated due to the fact that they are obedient to the influence of free water in their environment. Thus, adequate hydration of the body might be the best insurance against premature aging and an early loss of our different sensory systems.

MY ONGOING BATTLE WITH THE MEDICAL ESTABLISHMENT

It is the dawn of the twenty-first century, and yet I feel that the practice of medicine is becoming more and more regressive. Yes, people have learned that they are better off if they don't wait to get thirsty, and are taking measures to prevent their bodies from becoming dehydrated. They have learned that they feel better and are more energetic. They carry their water with them when they go out of the house; they take their water when they exercise; a vast majority are drinking water in preference to manufactured beverages and alcoholic drinks; schools are now getting wise to the harmful effect of sodas on children and are throwing out the vending machines. This has become a mandate in California, and other states are beginning to follow. Some researchers have found that children's scholastic performance dramatically improves when they drink water instead of the sodas they used to drink.

Yet all of a sudden an emeritus professor from Dartmouth Medical School publishes an article in the *American Journal of Physiology* saying he has not found any scientific reason why people should drink unless they are thirsty. The interesting part of all this is that this article was first posted on the Internet and released to the news agencies for its fast-track distribution before the paper version of the journal was published later in the year. The media from all over the world went to town on this orchestrated public-relations issue.

Realizing that this view, if allowed to stand, could potentially harm millions of trusting people from all over the world who might be influenced by the source of information, I wrote a brief scientific rebuttal to the published views and started disseminating the rebuttal. I have published the article on the Internet and it is now available for review by others. I am waiting for some reaction from the medical journals that received my rebuttal. I daresay, since my position is contrary to commercial interests of the sick-care system, no official reaction would be forthcoming. The article is presented below for those who might be interested in my logic; it is based on the new findings of molecular physiology of dehydration that you now understand.

You see why the information on water in this book is something you need to cherish. I don't believe you will get its benefits from the medical establishment in this country anytime soon.

Waiting to Get Thirsty Is to Die Prematurely and Very Painfully

Heinz Valtin, M.D., an emeritus professor at Dartmouth Medical School, has ventured the opinion that there is no scientific merit in drinking eight 8-ounce glasses of water a day and not waiting to get thirsty before correcting dehydration. This view, published in the *American Journal of Physiology*, August 2002, is the very foundation of all that is wrong with modern medicine, which is costing this nation $1.7 trillion a year, rising at the rate of 12 percent every year. Dr. Valtin's view, in my opinion, is as absurd as waiting for the final stages of a killer infection before giving the patient the appropriate antibiotics. His views are based on the erroneous assumption that dry mouth is an accurate sign of dehydration.

Like the colleagues he says he has consulted, Dr. Valtin does not seem to be aware of an important paradigm shift in medicine. All past views in medicine were based on the wrong assumption that it is the solutes in the body that regulate all functions and that the solvent has no direct role in any of the body's physiological functions. In medical schools it is taught that water is only a solvent, a packing material and a means of transport, that water has no metabolic function of its own. I have come across this level of ignorance about the primary physiological role of water at another Ivy League medical school from another eminent professor of physiology who, like Dr. Valtin, researched and taught the water-regulatory mechanisms of the kidney to medical students and doctors. Only when I asked him what "hydrolysis" is, did the penny drop and he admit the scientific fact that water is a nutrient and does indeed possess a dominant metabolic role in all physiological functions of the body.

Dr. Valtin's emphasis on the water-regulatory role of the kidneys limits his knowledge to the body's mechanisms of "deficit management" of the water needs of the body. He seems to base his views of thirst management of the body on the vital roles of vasopressin, the antidiuretic hormone, and the renin-angiotensin system, the elements that get engaged in the drought-management programs of the body, when the body has already become dehydrated. Indeed, he thinks dehydration is a state of the body when it loses 5 percent of its water content; and that one should wait until at some level of such water loss the urge to drink some kind of "fluid" will correct the water deficit in the body. This view might have seemed plausible twenty-five years ago. Today it exposes the tragic limitations of knowledge of the human physiology that is available to a prestigious medical school in America.

In his recently published and widely reported assertions, Dr. Valtin does not take into consideration the fact that water is a nutrient. Its vital "hydrolytic" role would be lost to all the physiological functions that would be affected by its shortage in its osmotically "free state." Another oversight is the fact that it is the interior of the cells of the body that would become drastically dehydrated. In dehydration, 66 percent of the water loss is from the interior of the cells, 26 percent of the loss is from extracellular fluid volume, and only 8 percent of the loss is borne by the blood tissue in the vascular system, which constricts within its network of capillaries and maintains the integrity of the circulation system.

Philippa M. Wiggin has shown that the mechanism that controls or brings about the effective function of the cation pumps utilizes the energy-transforming property of water, the solvent: "The source of energy for cation transport or ATP synthesis lies in increases in chemical potentials with increasing hydration of small cations and polyphosphate anions in the highly structured interfacial aqueous phase of the two phosphorylated intermediates." Waiting to get thirsty, when the body fluids become concentrated before thirst is induced, one loses the energy-generating properties of water in the dehydrated cells of the body. This is a major reason why we should prevent dehydration, rather than wait to correct it. This new understanding of the role of water in cation exchange is enough justification to let the body engage in prudent surplus-water management rather than forcing it into drought and deficit-water management, which is what Dr. Valtin is recommending people do.

In his research on the "conformational change in biological macromolecules," Ephraim Katchalski-Katzir of the Weizmann Institute of Science has shown that the "proteins and enzymes of the body function more efficiently in solutions of lower viscosity." Thus, water loss from the interior of the cells would adversely affect their efficiency of function. This finding alone negates Dr. Valtin's view that we should let dehydration get established before drinking water. Since it is desirable that all cells of the body should function efficiently within their physiological roles, it would be more prudent to optimally hydrate the body rather than wait for the drought-management programs of the body to induce thirst. Furthermore, it is much easier for the body to deal with a slight surplus of water than to suffer from its shortfall and have to ration and allocate water to vital organs at the expense of less vital functions of the body. The outcome of constantly circulating concentrated blood in the vascular system is truly an invitation to catastrophe.

The tragedy of waiting to get thirsty hits home when it is realized that the sharpness of thirst perception is gradually lost as we get older. Phillips and associates have shown that after twenty-four hours of water deprivation, the elderly still do not recognize they are thirsty: "The important finding is that despite their obvious physiologic need, the elderly subjects were not markedly thirsty." Bruce and associates have shown that between the ages of twenty and seventy, the ratio of water inside the cells to the amount of water outside the cells drastically changes from 1.1 to 0.8. Undoubtedly this marked change in the intracellular water balance would not take place if the osmotic push and pull of life could favor water diffusion through the cell membranes everywhere in the body—at the rate of 10^{-3} centimeters per second. Only by relying on the reverse osmotic process of expanding the extracellular water content of the body, so as to filter and inject "load-free" water into vital cells by the actions of vasopressin and the renin-angiotensin-aldosterone systems—when the body physiology is constantly forced to rely on its drought-management programs—could such a drastic change in the water balance of the body result.

Two other scientific discoveries are disregarded

when Dr. Valtin recommends people should wait until they get thirsty before they drink water. One, the initiation of the thirst mechanisms is not triggered by vasopressin and the renin-angiotensin systems—these systems are involved only in water conservation and forced hydration of the cells. Thirst is initiated when the Na^+-K^+-ATPase pump is inadequately hydrated. It is water that generates voltage gradient by adequately hydrating the pump proteins in the neurotransmission systems of the body. This is the reason the brain tissue is 85 percent water and cannot endure the level of "thirst-inducing" dehydration that is considered safe in the article published by Dr. Valtin.

Two, the missing piece of the scientific puzzle in the water-regulatory mechanisms of the body, which has been exposed since 1987, and which Dr. Valtin and his colleagues need to know, is the coupled activity of the neurotransmitter histamine to the efficiency of the cation exchange, its role in the initiation of the drought-management programs, and its role in the catabolic processes when the body is becoming more and more dehydrated. Based on the primary water-regulatory functions of histamine, and the active role of water in all physiologic and metabolic functions of the body—as the hydrolytic initiator of all solute functions—the symptoms of thirst are those produced by excess histamine activity and its subordinate mechanisms, which get engaged in the drought-management programs of the body. They include asthma, allergies, and the major pains of the body, such as heartburn, colitis pain, rheumatoid joint pain, back pain, migraine headaches, fibromyalgic pains, and even anginal pain. And since vasopressin and the renin-angiotensin-aldosterone activity in the body are subordinates to the activation of histamine, their role in raising the blood pressure is a part of the drought-management programs of the body. Their purpose of forced delivery of water into vital cells demands a greater injection pressure to counteract the direction of osmotic pull of water from inside the cells of the body when it is dehydrated.

From the new perspective of my twenty-two years of clinical and scientific research into molecular physiology of dehydration, and the peer-reviewed introduction of a paradigm shift in medical science, recognizing histamine as a neurotransmitter in charge of the water regulation of the body, I can safely say that the sixty million Americans with hypertension, the one hundred ten million with chronic pains, the fifteen million with diabetes, the seventeen million with asthma, the fifty million with allergies, the nearly one hundred million obese people in America, and more, all did exactly as Dr. Valtin recommends. They all waited to get thirsty. Had they realized water is a natural antihistamine and a more effective diuretic, I believe these people would have been saved the agony of their health problems.

References:
Batmanghelidj, F., M.D., "Pain: A Need for Paradigm Change," *Anticancer Research* 7, no. 5B (Sept.-Oct. 1987): 971–990. Full article posted on www.water-cure.com.

————. "Neurotransmitter Histamine: An Alternative View," *Book of Abstracts*, Third Interscience

World Conference on Inflammation, Analgesics and Immunomodulators, Monte-Carlo (March 1989): 37. The Abstract and the full article are posted on www.watercure.com.

————. *Your Body's Many Cries for Water*. Vienna, Va.: Global Health Solutions, Inc., 1995.

————. *ABC of Asthma, Allergies and Lupus*. Vienna, Va.: Global Health Solutions, Inc., 2000.

Bruce A., M. Anderson, B. Arvidsson, and B. Isacksson., "Body Composition, Predictions of Normal Body Potassium, Body Water and Body Fat in Adults on the Basis of Body Height, Body Weight and Age," *Scand. J Clin. Lab. Invest* 40 (1980): 461–473.

Katchalski-Katzir, Ephraim, "Conformational Changes in Biological Macromolecules." *Biorheology* 21(1984): 57–74.

Phillips, P. A., B. J. Rolls, J. G. G. Ledingham, M. L. Forsling, J. J. Morton, M. J. Crowe, and L. Wollner, "Reduced Thirst After Water Deprivation in Healthy Elderly Men," *The New England Journal of Medicine* 311, no. 12 (September 1985): 753–759.

Wiggins, P. M., "A Mechanism of ATP-Driven Cation Pumps," in *Biophysics of Water*, edited by Felix Franks and Sheila F. Mathis. West Sussex: John Wiley and Sons, Ltd.,1982.

CHAPTER 3

BASICS OF NEW MEDICINE FOR THE NEXT FEW THOUSAND YEARS

As I explained earlier, it is *water* (solvent) that regulates all the functions of the body, including the action of all the *solids* (solutes) that water carries around. This paradigm shift is a breakthrough in the fundamentals of medical science. This shift of attention is the key to a radically different approach to all disciplines of science in the future, including the basics of medicine and biochemistry. This new focus will ultimately change the structure of thought in research in any discipline of science.

What follows is a bird's-eye view of the scientific importance of this paradigm shift in medicine. It may take years before the profoundness of its ramifications can reach the public, but the change is unavoidable. The new paradigm can explain the cause of and show cures for so many "disease conditions" that it will make mainstream medicine of 2003 look ridiculous.

There are many reasons why we need to pay serious attention to our daily water intake. Here are some of them.

FORTY-SIX REASONS WHY YOUR BODY NEEDS WATER EVERY DAY

1. Without water, nothing lives.
2. Comparative shortage of water first suppresses and eventually kills some aspects of the body.
3. Water is the main source of energy—it is the "cash flow" of the body.
4. Water generates electrical and magnetic energy inside each and every cell of the body—it provides the power to live.
5. Water is the bonding adhesive in the architectural design of the cell structure.
6. Water prevents DNA damage and makes its repair mechanisms more efficient—less abnormal DNA is made.
7. Water increases greatly the efficiency of the immune system in the bone marrow, where the immune system is formed (all its mechanisms)—including its efficiency against cancer.
8. Water is the main solvent for all foods, vitamins, and minerals. It is used in the breakdown of food into smaller particles and their eventual metabolism and assimilation.
9. Water energizes food, and food particles are then able to supply the body with this energy during digestion. This is why food without water has absolutely no energy value for the body.
10. Water increases the body's rate of absorption of essential substances in food.
11. Water is used to transport all substances inside the body.

12. Water increases the efficiency of red blood cells in collecting oxygen in the lungs.
13. When water reaches a cell, it brings the cell oxygen and takes the waste gases to the lungs for disposal.
14. Water clears toxic waste from different parts of the body and takes it to the liver and kidneys for disposal.
15. Water is the main lubricant in the joint spaces and helps prevents arthritis and back pain.
16. Water is used in the spinal discs to make them "shock-absorbing water cushions."
17. Water is the best lubricating laxative and prevents constipation.
18. Water helps reduce the risk of heart attacks and strokes.
19. Water prevents clogging of arteries in the heart and the brain.
20. Water is essential for the body's cooling (sweat) and heating (electrical) systems.
21. Water gives us power and electrical energy for all brain functions, most particularly thinking.
22. Water is directly needed for the efficient manufacture of all neurotransmitters, including serotonin.
23. Water is directly needed for the production of all hormones made by the brain, including melatonin.
24. Water can help prevent attention deficit disorder in children and adults.
25. Water increases efficiency at work; it expands your attention span.
26. Water is a better pick-me-up than any other beverage in the world—and it has no side effects.
27. Water helps reduce stress, anxiety, and depression.
28. Water restores normal sleep rhythms.

29. Water helps reduce fatigue—it gives us the energy of youth.
30. Water makes the skin smoother and helps decrease the effects of aging.
31. Water gives luster and shine to the eyes.
32. Water helps prevent glaucoma.
33. Water normalizes the blood-manufacturing systems in the bone marrow—it helps prevent leukemia and lymphoma.
34. Water is absolutely vital for making the immune system more efficient in different regions to fight infections and cancer cells where they are formed.
35. Water dilutes the blood and prevents it from clotting during circulation.
36. Water decreases premenstrual pains and hot flashes.
37. Water and heartbeats create the dilution and waves that keep things from sedimenting in the bloodstream.
38. The human body has no stored water to draw on during dehydration. This is why you must drink regularly and throughout the day.
39. Dehydration prevents sex hormone production—one of the primary causes of impotence and loss of libido.
40. Drinking water separates the sensations of thirst and hunger.
41. To lose weight, water is the best way to go—drink water on time and lose weight without much dieting. Also, you will not eat excessively when you feel hungry but are in fact only thirsty for water.
42. Dehydration causes deposits of toxic sediments in the tissue spaces, joints, kidneys, liver, brain, and skin. Water will clear these deposits.

43. Water reduces the incidence of morning sickness in pregnancy.
44. Water integrates mind and body functions. It increases ability to realize goals and purpose.
45. Water helps prevent the loss of memory as we age. It helps reduce the risk of Alzheimer's disease, multiple sclerosis, Parkinson's disease, and Lou Gehrig's disease.
46. Water helps reverses addictive urges, including those for caffeine, alcohol, and some drugs.

SOME OF THE PRIMARY PROPERTIES AND FUNCTIONS OF WATER IN THE BODY

1. Water is the bulk material that fills empty spaces in the body.
2. Water is the vehicle of transport for the circulation of blood cells.
3. Water is a solvent for the materials that dissolve in it, including oxygen.
4. Water is the adhesive that binds solid parts of the cell together. Just as ice has a sticky effect, so water seems to become sticky at the cell membrane. It is responsible for holding things together and forming a membrane or protective barrier around the cell.
5. The neurotransmission systems of the brain and nerves depend on rapid movement of sodium and potassium in and out of the membrane along the full length of the nerves. Water that is loose and not bonded with something else is free to move across the cell membrane and turn the element-moving pumps.

6. Some of the element-moving pumps are voltage-generating pumps. Thus, efficiency of neurotransmission systems depends on the availability of free and unengaged water in the nerve tissues. In its osmotic urge to get into the cell, water generates energy by turning the pump units that force potassium into the cell and push sodium outside the cell—just as water turns the turbines at a hydroelectric dam to make electricity. Up to now, however, it has been assumed that all energy storage in adenosine triphosphate (ATP)—the substance that "burns" and gives out "heat" to "cook" any of the chemical reactions required for the cell to function—is from food intake. This is why water has not received much attention as a source of energy in the energy-generating systems in the body.

7. Water is the central regulator of energy and osmotic balance in the body. Sodium and potassium stick to the protein of the pump and act as the "magnet of the dynamo" when water rotates the pump proteins. The rapid turn of these cation (pronounced *cat-i-on*) pumps generates energy that is stored at many different locations in three different pool types.

ATP is one type of energy pool. Another energy storage pool is guanosine triphosphate (GTP). A third system is in the endoplasmic reticulum that captures and traps calcium. For every two units of calcium that are trapped, the energy equivalent of one unit of ATP is stored in the connection of the two calcium atoms. For every two units of calcium that are separated from one another and released, one unit of energy—to make a new unit of ATP—is also released. This mechanism of calcium entrapment as a means of energy storage makes the bone structure of the body not only its scaffolding but also its Fort Knox—like investment of your cash in gold reserve. Hence, when there is severe dehydration— and consequently a decreased supply of hydroelectric energy—the body taps into the bones for their stored energy. Thus, I believe that the primary cause of osteoporosis is persistent dehydration.

8. The foods we eat are the products of energy conversion from the initial electrical-energy-generating property of water. All living and growing species, humans included, survive as a result of energy generation from water. One major problem in the scientific evaluation of the body is the lack of understanding of the magnitude of our body's dependence on energy from hydroelectricity.

9. The electricity produced at the cell membrane also forces the nearby proteins to align themselves and get ready for their chemical reactions.

Blood is normally about 94 percent water when the body is fully hydrated (red cells are actually "water bags" that contain the colored hemoglobin). Inside the cells of the body, there should ideally be about 75 percent water. Because of this difference in water levels outside and inside the cells, an osmotic flow of water into the cells normally occurs. There are hundreds of thousands of voltage-generating pump units at the cell membranes, much like the turbines used in hydroelectric dams. The water that flows through them rotates these pumps. This rush of water creates hydroelectric energy. At the same time, and as part of the same process, elements such as sodium and potassium are exchanged.

Only water that is free and can move about—the water you drink—generates hydroelectric energy at the cell membrane. The previously supplied water that is now busy with other functions cannot leave its binding position to rush elsewhere. This is why water by itself should be considered the most suitable pick-me-up beverage and should be consumed at regular intervals during the day. The good thing about water as a source of energy is the fact that any excess water is passed out of the body. It manufactures the needed energy to top up the reserves in the cells and then leaves the body (carrying with it the toxic waste of the cells). It is not stored.

When there is dehydration because a person is not drinking enough water, the cells become depleted of their ready energy. They then have to depend more on energy generation from food that is consumed instead of water. In this situation, the body is pushed into storing fat and using its protein and starch reserves, because it is easier to break these elements down than the stored fat. This is the reason why 37 percent of people in America are grossly overweight. Their bodies are engaged in perpetual crisis management of dehydration.

The word *hydrolysis* (loosening, dissolving, breaking, or splitting by the participating action of water) is used when water becomes involved in the metabolism of other materials. Activities that depend on hydrolysis include the breakdown of a protein into the different amino acids that have been used to make that particular protein, and the breakdown of large fatty particles into smaller fatty acid units. Without water, hydrolysis cannot take place. It follows, then, that the hydrolytic function of water also constitutes the metabolism of water itself. What this means is that water itself needs to be broken down first—hydrolyzed—before the body can use the various components in food. This is why we need to supply the body with water before we eat solid foods.

CHAPTER 4

WATER REGULATION OF A FETUS
AND AN INFANT

From the very moment of conception, when the father's sperm fuses with the mother's egg to form a single-cell unit of life, that cell has to divide, and divide, and divide millions of times over to develop into a form that can firmly connect itself to the uterine wall. By the time it grows to be a full-term baby, about a trillion cell divisions will have taken place. For this to happen, it has to impose a water-regulatory pattern for its needs on the mother's water-intake systems. Remember, each new cell that forms has to be filled up mainly with water. All of a sudden, the mother has to take in more water to supply the growing demands of the child. Even when the child is born, the mother has to provide the water needs of the infant through her milk-manufacturing system. The mother's breast is both a sort of water fountain for her child and a source of food.

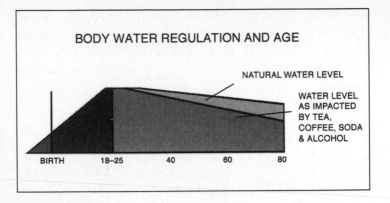

Figure 4.1: A graphic model of the proposed body-water regulation at the three major phases of life: the fetus, the growing child, and the fully developed person, using water versus dehydrating fluids.

Early-Pregnancy Morning Sickness

In light of the above information, how does a pregnant woman register her new level of water needs? I am going to share with you a secret that has never before been recognized. The early-pregnancy morning sickness of a pregnant woman is a most meaningful thirst signal. In fact, it is the very first sign of dehydration of the mother and fetus together. It is brought about by the water-regulatory action of histamine.

This indication of the water needs of the growing fetus through the mother's sensory system is an important signal that connects the child's sensory system for its water needs to the mother's regulatory mechanisms. Most mothers adjust their water intake by the third month and the morning sickness disappears, but some don't and continue to live a life that promotes dehydration in the fetus as well as themselves. The consequences can be catastrophic.

When a mother continues to drink coffee, tea, and alcohol during her pregnancy and does not take sufficient water, she influences the physiological pattern of the developing child in her uterus. The child draws the necessary ingredients for growth from the mother's pool of resources. The desperately needed ingredients include water, oxygen, and the amino acids that are available in the mother's circulation. Thus, the level of water intake and the composition of the amino acids made available during intrauterine life determine the assets of the growing child for natural development. These, in turn, establish a metering system that regulates the child's future growth and development.

The importance of the role of the mother's lifestyle during the physiological development of the child in the uterus is not fully realized. The mother is responsible for the creation of a healthy, natural chemical environment in which the child can grow through all the necessary developmental stages from a single cell to a full-term baby.

As we will learn later, the physiology and the chemical commands of stress in the body translate into an immediate adaptive and coping process to anticipated dehydration. Dehydration itself causes the body severe stress. The body establishes certain physiological and hormonal reactions to stress. The fetus is not protected from the physiological signals associated with the stresses of the mother. The indicators of stress that influence the mother's physiology and become the basis for her adaptive behavior also register with the child.

We should remember that all recordings of the mother's physiology are determined by chemical messenger systems. The influences of one or another transmitter system that becomes engaged in the stress-coping process of the mother can possibly affect the fetus. They will possibly create chemical readings in the child similar to those that are designed to be established in the mother.

Simply put, let us not underestimate the influence and responsibility of the mother for providing a normal chemical environment for the development, well-being, and future normal behavior of the fetus growing in her uterus—the preparatory school of life. The child's learning during its intrauterine "school days" can become the format settings for behavior and mood patterns in adult phases of life. Every form of behavior and thought translates into the release of a combination of chemical messenger systems. The release of chemical combinations can also code the brain of a growing fetus in the uterus. Thus, the lifestyle of a pregnant woman can influence the chemistry of a developing fetus. If she develops an imbalance in her chemistry, her fetus has to cope with the imbalance, too. It is true that the placenta acts as a selective barrier, but certain natural chemicals of the body go across the barrier, even in disproportionate amounts if these are present in the mother.

In short, the mother's range of chemistry is a template for the development of her child.

Similarly, a mother who consumes an excess of alcohol during pregnancy may produce a mentally fractured and unable-to-cope child. A developing brain needs much water. One of the ways of getting water through the cell wall is by the creation of small "showerhead" perforations that allow only water through. Other solid substances that are dissolved in the serum do not get into the cell when water is injected into the cell. The act of producing these very small perforations in the cell wall to let only water in is under the control of a hormone called vasopressin— the agent engaged in the drought-management program of the body.

Alcohol has been shown to prevent vasopressin formation and its functions. When alcohol consumption by the mother prevents the secretion and the needed actions of vasopressin, the same effect is produced in the child. The mother's brain structure is already formed, but the fetus's is not. The lack of vasopressin can result in the child's brain not developing normally. The child's lungs may also develop with abnormalities that could lead to cystic deformation. Because of the vital role of water in regulating all functions of the body, it is not accurate to blame most developmental abnormalities entirely on DNA malformation, as has been the case up to now. Dehydration could be a contributing factor.

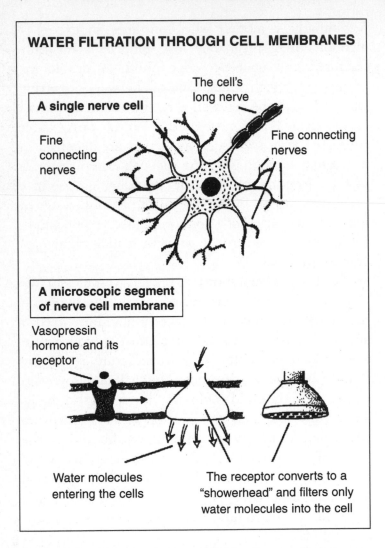

WATER FILTRATION THROUGH CELL MEMBRANES

A single nerve cell

The cell's long nerve

Fine connecting nerves

Fine connecting nerves

A microscopic segment of nerve cell membrane

Vasopressin hormone and its receptor

Water molecules entering the cells

The receptor converts to a "showerhead" and filters only water molecules into the cell

Figure 4.2: The schematic model of a nerve cell, its membrane wall, and the vasopressin receptor that becomes transformed into a type of "showerhead" that lets only water through its very small perforations. This is part of the mechanism of reverse osmosis that the body employs to deliver filtered water into vital cells.

Crib Death

Crib death/cot death (CD) or sudden infant death syndrome (SIDS) is the name given to the unexplainable and unpredictable death of a child in its crib. Losing an infant during its sleep is one of the most devastating tragedies imaginable. Every year, seven thousand to eight thousand babies between a few days and a year old die inexplicably while asleep. The greatest frequency is among infants two to six months old. Diagnosis relies on exclusion of other causes and is based on autopsy examination.

Vomiting up milk and then choking on it is usually not the cause of death. It is not caused by infections or colds. It is not the result of a contagious disease. The primary cause of CD is not really known.

I have thought much about the possible physiological events that might cause the death of an infant during sleep. I feel that the only plausible event that might be responsible, from the perspective of the paradigm shift, is the constriction of bronchioles due to dehydration and heat-management programs of the body, when the infant is possibly bundled too much and the room is warmer than it should be. I would call it *infantile asthma*. If childhood asthma can kill a few thousand annually, even when treatment is available, why should asthma not be considered as a primary cause of death in infants who have no means of expression when in deep sleep?

The formula milk the infant drinks may also contribute to CD. There is a marked difference between human milk and cow's milk. Cow's milk is more concentrated and has more fat and proteins than human milk. Cow's milk is designed for the needs of a calf that stands and begins to move and runs around in the first hour of life. The newborn child is immobile for the first several months of life. Herein lies the reason for the difference between the natural consistency and design of human milk and those of cow's milk. When cow's milk is formulated and given to infants as their only source of water—often parents are told not to give infants water—the metabolic system of the infant is burdened by digestion of the concentrated milk. Concentrated milk can have detrimental effects.

I was told at a medical conference that autopsies of infants who had died in car accidents showed an obvious partial blockage of the coronary arteries of those on formula milk, and *not* of those who were breast-fed. This is a significant revelation that has not been dealt with publicly and openly. I am of the opinion that the coronary arteries of infants on formula get blocked because the formulated milk composition is more concentrated than the mother's milk.

The normal practice is that the infant is given concentrated milk and bundled to sleep. While asleep, much water, in comparison to the weight of the infant, is lost from the lungs during the exhalation phase of the breathing process. This water loss from the lungs, on top of the fact that the milk contained possibly only just enough water for the digestion of the milk itself, leaves the infant's body short of water and forces it into physiological events for drought management. These include the secretion of increased amounts of histamine, which in infants is also a growth hormone and is abundantly available. Histamine is also a constrictor of bronchioles. It is possible that a certain combination of milk intake, unfavorable environmental conditions, and the inability to cool down could tip the balance toward the constriction of the bronchioles in the infant and cause silent death in sleep.

What surprises me is how the body of an infant is so resilient and adaptive that this problem is not seen more frequently. I can only think that the digestive process in the infant is so strongly active that the metabolic process manufactures some water from the breakdown of the solids in the milk to help the process in the same cycle of milk intake. If this is the case, what tips the balance against the infant and causes CD to occur are unfavorable environmental factors of too much heat and excessive covering of the body.

I think we should go back to the practice of introducing water into the diet of infants, particularly in the second to sixth months of life, when the occurrence of crib death is most frequent. They should not get too much of it, but a balanced amount and always with or after milk. This practice might cultivate a taste for water from infancy and establish a stronger thirst sensation—and prevent overeating when people really are only thirsty—later in life.

WATER REGULATION DURING CHILDHOOD AND ADOLESCENCE

When a child is born, its water needs for healthy growth and development are supplied initially by water in the milk it drinks, and then by water intake itself. The growth hormone and other water regulators drive the thirst mechanism and the body's calls for water. At the same time, the body retains water at any cost. The kidneys begin to concentrate the urine and draw as much water as possible away from the final stages of urine formation. The driving forces behind water regulation for growth are the growth hormone and other associated hormones and neurotransmitters, such as histamine.

Because they are growing, children are constantly and naturally dehydrated. The process of cell expansion and division uses up a great deal of water. Seventy-five percent of each cell is water. The body of a growing child constantly needs and calls for water; otherwise growth would not be possible. If the natural calls of the body for water are satisfied by manufactured chemical-containing fluids and sugar-containing drinks, healthy growth and development—events that water itself initiates—may not take place efficiently, and crisis events such as asthma and allergies may occur. Children and young adults should learn to drink water by itself and not substitute other beverages. The brain's alertness and learning capacity are proportionately dependent on the water intake of the individual. When teenagers, who should be alert and full of life, put their heads on the desk and fall asleep in class with a soda can next to them, it could be a sign that their bodies are short of water. Brain functions improve when water intake is increased to fully hydrate the body at all times.

I once had the occasion to lecture to three science

classes at a local high school. I checked the urine bowls in the toilet for the color of the morning urine passed by the male students. All the bowls contained very dark, obviously concentrated, urine—an indication of severe dehydration. Parents should become aware of the volume of water their children drink. It is their responsibility to educate their children about the importance of water, and to discourage addiction to manufactured colored drinks. This is not the statement of a puritan; it is based on an understanding of science.

WATER MANAGEMENT IN ADULTS

After full physical growth has taken place and the body is no longer in its growing phase of physical development, the effect of the growth hormone is no longer a dominant factor in the regulation of the body's water intake. At this stage of life, the body's water regulation becomes the primary responsibility of nerve centers in the brain that employ histamine as the chemical messenger.

It is at this phase of life that the thirst sensation becomes insufficient to regulate for adequate water intake. The reason for this failing thirst sensation seems to be very delicate, but simple. Our bodies, although many millions of years down the road of development from the earlier species that stepped out of water and ventured onto land, still depend on the same adaptive processes that were developed by their water-dwelling progenitors. They formed strong water-management systems to enable them to stay out of water for longer and longer periods. Although the body does not possess any means of retaining excess and spare water in the same way that fat is stored, it still has to be able to cope with periods of drought.

The physiology of the body is always dependent on water. Management of drought does not mean that the body cells become independent of water. It only means that certain areas of the body that are less in demand and not used all the time will be given survival rations only. The entry of water into these cells will not be by free flow, but will be coupled to the need-to-act commands to the cell. Water intake is regulated by a decreased flow of circulation to the inactive area. Then, if the area is forced into activity, the vascular (circulatory) system opens up and water is brought to the region.

From the age of about eighteen to twenty-five, when the body has reached full height and breadth, our regulation of water intake depends on the thirst sensation and our attempts at satisfying this sensation. Unfortunately, our thirst sensation, as it is understood today—a dry mouth—is not an accurate indicator of the body's actual water needs. If we don't feel thirsty, we tend not to drink water. We wait to become thirsty before we even begin to think of drinking water. The whole problem of health deterioration begins by this very attitude toward water intake—deficit management only—and even that is only in half measures. By the time the body reflects its thirst through invoking its thirst sensation, it is short of two to three glasses of water. We may drink only one glass, leaving the body with two glasses less than it needs. Unfortunately, this gap expands as we grow older.

REDUCTION OF THIRST SENSATION

The body has an ability to adapt to some hardship. Low food intake and temporary shortage of water in the body seem to invoke an adaptive process. The essential functions of the body are managed until we have access to food and water. In this process, the sensation of thirst can be confused with the feeling of hunger, because both sensations are similar in the way they register—they stem from low energy levels in the brain. This is one of the main contributing factors in the development of obesity in the young and the old. They mistakenly eat food to satisfy their thirst sensation.

They seem to respond to both calls—thirst and hunger—as if they are only hungry. They begin to eat until the thirst sensation gathers greater strength as a result of the additional load of solid food within the system, and only then do they drink some water. This type of thirst satisfaction is not enough for the urgent needs of the body, but is just enough to fall inside the body's limit of temporary adaptation to water shortage. In this way, the water shortage in the body becomes a steadily expanding chronic state, and new thresholds of adaptation are forced on the body. This process results in a slowly deteriorating loss of thirst sensation, so much so that the need for regular water intake as a sensation gradually becomes forgotten.

Histamine can act as a temporary substitute for water by releasing energy for some extremely sensitive body functions. In this way, the body can survive some dehydration. It seems the body begins to rely on the emergency functions of histamine and allows dehydration to continue. Still, no matter how useful the possession of these emergency powers, dehydration is damaging to some less-used functions of the body. Gradually establishing chronic dehydration produces constant changes, initially in the physiology and eventually in the chemistry of the body. The body begins to survive on the constant verge of failure.

The histamine-operated centers of the brain seem to recognize the levels of water that enter the body. If sufficient water enters the body, the active histamine centers gradually become disengaged from their full-time responsibility as water regulators. The engagement of histamine in drought management and its substitution for some energy-transforming functions of water decrease and are eventually phased out. It seems that the body begins to realize there is no water shortage and becomes more alert to and conscious of its calls for water—it begins to understand and manifest thirst. It seems to me that *the loss of the thirst sensation is an adaptive process to false information that water is not available because we don't drink it.*

If the body is once again conditioned to regular and adequate water intake, however, the thirst sensation becomes sharp and the urge to drink water becomes strong. The body begins to indicate water shortage more forcefully. The rehydration of the cells takes place slowly. The cells of the body are just like sponges—they get soaked slowly. Do not imagine the body will become optimally hydrated after just the first glass or two of water. The water that is taken will not immediately enter all the cells. Upon regular and adequate intake of water, the process of full hydration of the cells will take a few days. Only when you realize what damage dehydration can cause will you take seriously the need for strict adherence to hydrating the body regularly and well. The quantity and timing of water intake is very important and will be discussed in a later chapter.

Everyone knows water is essential. What is not fully realized is what happens when the body is not provided with adequate water on a regular basis. Also, what is meant by "the body begins to survive on the constant verge of failure"?

The human body is a composite structure made of many different systems. All these systems are dependent on the various properties of water for their normal function. When there is not enough water in the body for all the functions to take place, something has to give. When the body is only just managing to cope with daily routine activities and then a sudden emergency situation arises and an action has to take place, how will the body show its limitations? Suppose the body is in equilibrium within a threshold, and all of a sudden new obligations are thrust on it until the threshold is passed. How will the body show its shortfalls? In short, how will the body cope with the sudden stress of having to cope with emergency situations that demand water-dependent responses, when the body is already dehydrated? In essence, the answer to this question is the main topic of this book.

The damage of dehydration is established when the proteins and enzymes of the body become gradually, but increasingly, inefficient. The individual cells in the zone of dehydration begin to function less efficiently until eventually the loss of cell function becomes permanent. In any state of free-water loss from the body, 66 percent is lost from the cell content, 26 percent is lost from the fluid between the cells, and only 8 percent is lost from the blood volume. This causes concern in light of research by Bruce and associates. They have shown that as we grow older, from the ages of twenty to seventy, the water content inside the cells becomes less than the amount of water outside the cells of the body. The water inside the cells is gradually lost until the osmotic balance is reversed. This reversal of balance makes it gradually more difficult for our cells to absorb and hold water as we get older. The question we need to ask ourselves is: What happens to our bodies when they are allowed to undergo such a drastic transformation of their cell water content and composition? Read on for the answer.

CHAPTER 5

WHAT IS CHRONIC DEHYDRATION?

Imagine a juicy plum picked from the tree and left exposed to the sun or wind—it becomes a prune. The dehydration of the plum produces the shriveled interior and wrinkled skin that are typical of a drying fruit. Loss of water causes the internal and external structures of living things to change, be that dehydration in a fruit or in a person.

There are up to one hundred trillion cells in the body of a human being. Depending on the area where the dehydration has settled most, the cells in that region begin to wrinkle, and their inner functions are affected. A shortage of water in any region is reflected by different signals that denote dehydration and are the body's indicators of its local or general thirst. At present, these indicators of dehydration of the body, some of which I listed in a previous chapter, are not understood and are treated as indicators of disease conditions of unknown origin.

IDENTIFYING DEHYDRATION

- What are the common indicators of dehydration?
- What happens to our bodies when we don't drink enough water?
- What is "enough" water?

We now need to find the answer to these three important questions. A must-do before we begin: You need to turn on your brain's logic powers and put aside any preconceived ideas you might have. Whatever you have read about health matters in the past probably did not reflect the true importance of water to health and well-being.

From my perspective, there are three different sets of sensations that signal local or general thirst. At most of these stages, the presenting symptoms are reversible without much damage.

1. The General Perceptive "Feelings"

They include feeling tired, feeling flushed, feeling irritable, feeling anxious, feeling dejected, feeling depressed, not sleeping well, feeling heavy-headed, having irresistible cravings, and having a fear of crowds and leaving the house. Some of these will be discussed in the next chapter.

2. The Drought-Management Programs

The second group of conditions that represent indicators of dehydration are the body's drought- and resource-management programs. There are five distinct conditions that denote states of dehydration and operative rationing processes that can be corrected easily. The sixth in this group consists of a number of conditions that have been classified as autoimmune diseases, but should be looked at as a sort of cannibalistic process of resource management at the expense of the body's own tissues brought about by persistent dehydration. The conditions are:

1. Asthma
2. Allergies
3. Hypertension
4. Constipation
5. Type II diabetes
6. Autoimmune diseases

3. The More Drastic Emergency Indicators of Local Dehydration

After much clinical and scientific research, my understanding is this: Depending on the location of acid buildup inside the cells, the following forms of pain are early indicators of potential genetic damage produced by chronic dehydration in the human body:

1. Heartburn
2. Dyspeptic pain
3. Anginal pain
4. Lower back pain
5. Rheumatoid joint pains, including ankylosing spondylitis
6. Migraine headaches
7. Colitis pain
8. Fibromyalgic pains
9. Bulimia
10. Morning sickness during pregnancy

There is a further set of conditions that represent complications, tissue transformation, and organ damage caused by persistent dehydration in the fourth dimension, time. Each of these conditions will be explained thoroughly in upcoming chapters.

CHAPTER 6

NEWLY RECOGNIZED THIRST PERCEPTIONS

The following are perceptive feelings (some of which are labeled "psychological disorders") that I believe signal dehydration:

1. *Feeling tired without a plausible reason.* Water is the main source of energy formation in the body. Even the food that is supposed to be a good source of energy has no value to the body until it is hydrolyzed by water and energized in the process. Furthermore, the energy source for neurotransmission and for the operational directives that get things done is hydroelectricity, which is formed in the nerve pathways and their connection to the muscles and joints in the body.
2. *Feeling flushed.* When the body is dehydrated, and the brain cannot draw sufficient water from the circulation to satisfy its needs, it commands a proportionate dilation of the blood vessels that reach it. Furthermore, the face is not a simple organ that supports two eyes, a mouth, a nose, and two ears. It

is a receptor dish with an abundant supply of nerve endings that constantly monitor the environment and report their information to the brain. In other words, the face is an extension of the brain with highly sensitive functions. Its nerve endings need to be hydrated, too; hence the increased circulation to the face at the same time as the brain gets its increased blood supply. If you see someone with a red nose and flushed face—often seen in alcoholics, because alcohol truly dehydrates the brain, leading to hangover headaches—that person is dehydrated and in need of water.

3. *Feeling irritable and unreasonably short-tempered.* Irritability is a copout process so as not to engage in a brain-energy-consuming involvement beyond that particular moment. Give irritable people a couple of glasses of water and you will see them calm down and become fairly amiable.

4. *Feeling anxious.* This is a perceptive way in which the frontal part of the brain can reflect its concern over water shortage in its domain of activity. I cannot imagine a more eloquent way for the thinking brain to reflect its anxiety about dehydration in the body of its delinquent owner. Obviously, when the body wanted water, it must have been given other beverages that did not satisfy its real needs.

5. *Feeling dejected and inadequate.* The capital assets of any body are its essential amino acid reserves. These types of amino acids are used in so many different functions, including for neurotransmission,

that their shortage in the body means loss of assets that the brain assesses as insufficient and inadequate for its undertakings. Dehydration depletes some of these amino acids incessantly, and this shortage triggers a feeling of dejection.

6. *Feeling depresssed.* This heralds a more serious phase of dehydration, in which the body, in the absence of water, has to use up some of its vital assets as antioxidants to cope with the toxic waste of metabolism that has not been cleared by sufficient production of urine. These assets include the amino acids tryptophan (pronounced *trip-toh-fan*) and tyrosine, which are sacrificed in the liver as antioxidants to neutralize toxic waste. For the manufacture of serotonin, melatonin, tryptamine, and indolamine, the brain uses tryptophan; all of these elements are vital neurotransmitters that are used to balance and integrate body functions. If they are inadequate in the body, depression sets in. Tyrosine is another amino acid that the brain uses to manufacture adrenaline, noradrenaline, and dopamine, which are the "go-getter" neurotransmitters. Their insufficient activity will ground a person into inactivity and a sorrowful state of mind.

As I was editing this book, an article on depression in the *Washington Post* of Tuesday, May 7, 2002, revealed a deep-rooted deception by the pharmaceutical industry. Headlined AGAINST DEPRESSION, A SUGAR PILL IS HARD TO BEAT, the article exposes how the drug industry has bent the truth in clinical trials to show an edge in favor of Prozac, Paxil, and Zoloft, whereas a simple sugar pill—placebo—produced more positive results in relieving depression. This article surmises that the splendid results of the sugar pill against the much-touted drugs could be because, in the clinical trials, the subjects received much more attention and care than a depressed person who visits the doctor for a few minutes a month. It seems there is an infinitely greater healing power within a person who is cared for. In medicine there used to be a dictum, now forgotten—"The duty of a doctor is to amuse the patient while nature heals." Doctors have to show empathy to their patients.

Now that I am addressing the role of water in emotional problems, let me quote from a reader review of my book *Your Body's Many Cries for Water*, posted on the Barnes & Noble Web site, www.bn.com. M. S. writes: "'Water' has made a difference in my life." It seems that M. S. had been diagnosed with mild manic depression and had been given lithium for four to five years. He says he started on water and salt and some vitamins, according to the instructions in the book, and within two months he was able to stop taking his lithium. He had been visiting his doctors for nine years without significant improvement, and now writes, "My LIFE has been truly ENHANCED from reading the book."

7. *Feeling heavy-headed.* This is the sign that the brain is commanding more circulation for its needs. It

could be the heralding sensation for a migraine headache that may ensue if the increased blood flow to the brain does not result in adequate hydration of the brain cells. Do not forget that the brain cells, in their constant activity, produce toxic waste of metabolism, which must be cleared at all times. The brain cells cannot endure a buildup of acidic materials in their interior environment. The initial heaviness felt in the head could reflect this phase of brain physiology.

8. *Disturbed sleep, particularly in the elderly.* The body will not have a restful night's sleep if it is short of water. A full eight hours' sleep will further dehydrate the body because much water is lost in respiration and possible perspiration under heavy bedcovers. If the body receives water and a little salt, sleep rhythm will be reestablished immediately. The following letter is from a man who found my Water Cure program instrumental in relieving many problems, including an interrupted sleep pattern. His story highlights a number of the perceptive symptoms of dehydration I have pointed out already.

My name is D. H. and I was turned on to your Web site by a friend on the Internet. Firstly, I read much of what is on your Web site and have been impressed by the content. In fact, I opened a chatroom on paltalk devoted to directing people to your site and discussing the benefits of drinking water with salt. I have been on The Water Cure for about three weeks now and I can definitely say I'm feeling better. My blood pressure is lower and my heart rate is around 58. I seem to sleep better at night and I have better energy level during the day. Also, I have a peaceful feeling now and seem to worry less. All in all it has been a positive experience. I thank you for promoting The Water Cure and I have joined your bandwagon to spread the good word. Thanks again for helping others unselfishly. D. H.

9. *Anger and quick temper.* These more expressive ways of showing dehydration were explained in section 3 under the heading Feeling Irritable.

10. *Unreasonable impatience.* Maintaining your patience to stay on a course or an assignment is an energy-consuming undertaking for the brain. If it doesn't have a sufficient stored reserve of energy, it has to put an end to the undertaking as quickly as possible. This process of quick disengagement is labeled "impatience." Don't forget, water manufactures hydroelectric energy at a rate that can replenish the used-up amount. Energy from food has to go through many steps of molecular conversion until it is stored in the energy pools in the cells. Even this process needs water for hydrolysis to make the components of food usable as sources of energy.

11. *Very short attention span.* This is another disengagement process for the brain that needs energy to focus on a topic or a learning process. The more

hydrated the brain, the more energy it can manufacture to imprint new information in its memory banks. Attention deficit disorder in children is similarly produced by dehydration when children choose sodas as their preferred drinks.

12. *Shortness of breath in an otherwise healthy person without lung disease or infection.* People who want to exercise without feeling short of breath should drink water before they exert themselves in any form of physical activity.

13. *Cravings for manufactured beverages such as coffee, tea, sodas, and alcoholic drinks.* This is the way your brain tells you that you need to be hydrated. These cravings are based on a condition reflex that associates hydration with the intake of these beverages, which actually dehydrate the body further. The process of continuous dehydration is stressful and causes the brain to secrete stress hormones, which include endorphins—the natural opiates of the body that help it get through its environmental crisis. One of the reasons why people continue drinking these beverages is their increasing addiction to the level of their own endorphin production. This is why caffeine and alcohol are addictive substances and cause withdrawal symptoms. The next stage to this kind of addiction could be the use of harder drugs that put a constant drive on endorphin secretion by the body. Thus, if children are to be directed toward a drug-free form of life, it should start with eliminating caffeine from their diets.

14. *Dreaming of oceans, rivers, or other bodies of water* is a form of subconsciously generated association to reach a source of water to quench thirst. The brain has a tendency to simulate an experience in order to give instructions to the person to perform a function, even in deep sleep.

There is usually some significance to dreams. I will never forget a dream I had when I was a house doctor working at St. Mary's Hospital Medical School in London. At the time, I was responsible for the daily care of thirty acute beds (as they were known) in a very active surgical unit of the hospital. I could never get more than three or four hours of sleep at night. Naturally, when my head hit the pillow in those days, I slept like the dead. On one of those busy days, I reached my lunch late and had to eat it many hours after it was cooked. It was a plate of crayfish and some vegetables.

I was too busy to feel any discomfort after eating the food. I went to bed in the early hours of the morning and all but died in bed. Not long into my sleep, I started to dream that I was in a boat on rough seas. The boat was being thrown about, up and down and side to side, motions dictated by the choppy sea. I started feeling more and more nauseated until I could no longer hold down what I had eaten, and only just managed to reach the sink in my room to throw up the food that had obviously gone bad. My brain could not have translated my need to get up and get rid of the contents of my stomach any other way. It could only prepare me by exposing me to associated thoughts around nausea and vomiting. What better way than to take me through a sort of dry-run experience of sea-sickness?

CHAPTER 7

THE PRIMARY DROUGHT- AND RESOURCE-MANAGEMENT PROGRAMS

From the vantage point of the new medical science, the following conditions should be considered labels placed on the physiological processes in the body that denote a form of rationing and resource management when there is a limited supply of free water and other primary elements in the body:

1. Asthma
2. Allergies
3. Hypertension, or high blood pressure
4. Type II diabetes
5. Constipation
6. Autoimmune diseases

If you don't drink water regularly every day of your life, and don't understand the significance of pain, shortness of breath, and allergies as signs of dehydration, you will force your body into a disease state. Any of the above conditions will herald the beginnings of body decay produced by local or general water shortage and the associated chemical environmental changes.

Reversal of autoimmune conditions is not easy and not always possible. To reverse them requires an in-depth understanding of the importance of the acid–alkaline balance and the metabolic aspects associated with dehydration, such as the loss of a range of amino acids, insufficient absorption or loss of vital minerals like zinc and magnesium, and the absolute need for essential vitamins and fatty acids.

ASTHMA AND ALLERGIES

What is asthma? It is said people have asthma when they become short of breath, without any warning, to the point of nearly suffocating. Several thousand people die from suffocation due to asthma every year. Sometimes the onset of asthma is associated with repeated dry coughs with each breath. There is always an associated wheezing when exhaling, without an apparent infection in the lungs. Asthma affects more than seventeen million Americans, mostly children. I believe that asthma and allergies are the body's crisis calls for water. *They denote a state of dehydration in the human body. They herald continuing degeneration of the body until other complications of dehydration get established and can cause early death.*

My experience and research tell me that the body possesses a number of highly sophisticated emergency thirst signals. We need to be aware of these newly identified indicators of water shortage in our body. All you may need to do to cure some of your health problems is drink water instead of other fluids.

Question: What has all this got to do with asthma?

Answer: Asthma and allergy—conditions mainly treated with different kinds of antihistamine medications—are important indicators of dehydration in the body. Histamine is an important neurotransmitter that primarily regulates the thirst mechanism, for increased water intake. It also establishes a system of rationing for the available water in the drought-stricken body. Histamine is a most noble element employed in drought management of the body. It is not the villain that we have been led to believe due to our limitation of knowledge about the human body.

In dehydration, histamine production and its activity increase greatly, and this generates the emergency thirst signals and indicators of the water-rationing program that is taking place. Increased histamine release in the lungs causes spasms of the bronchioles, making them constrict. This natural spasmodic action of histamine on the bronchial tubes is part of the design of the body to conserve water that normally evaporates during breathing—the winter "steam."

In dehydration, lung tissue becomes very vulnerable. The air sacs in the lungs have very thin walls and need water to keep them moist at all times. The constant flow of air through these sacs also evaporates the available water in their lining. Dehydration automatically reduces the amount of available water

---

in these tissues and causes damage, unless the rate of airflow is reduced. In essence, this is the rationale behind the blockage of airflow through the lungs in asthmatics. Histamine is responsible for cutting down the rate of airflow through the lungs. It causes constriction of the bronchioles that are attached to the air sacs. Histamine also stimulates the production of added amounts of thick and viscous mucus that partially plug the bronchioles and protect the lining of the bronchioles themselves. All these actions of histamine in dehydration are carried out to protect the delicate passageways of the body that are in direct contact with the outside air and could easily become dried up and parched if not protected.

Histamine will be further discussed in the section on neurotransmitters in chapter 10.

ALLERGIES AND THE IMMUNE SYSTEM

When we become dehydrated, histamine sees to it that the available water in the body is well preserved and distributed according to a priority of function. The rate of histamine production in the body increases exponentially when the body becomes more and more dehydrated.

Supplying the body with water causes a disappearance of histamine from areas where it should not be present. With adequate water supply, histamine production, and its excess release, is inhibited proportionately. This relationship of water to histamine has been demonstrated in several animal experiments. It is now physiologically apparent that water by itself has very strong natural antihistaminic properties.

Immune System Suppression

There are certain white cells that are sensitive to histamine and that strongly inhibit the activity of the immune system in the bone marrow. There are twice as many of these white cells as there are cells that stimulate the immune system. Thus, dehydration that can cause the production and release of more than a certain amount of histamine may, in the long run, suppress the immune systems of the body at its central command station, the bone marrow.

Since there is a greater-than-normal rate of histamine production and storage in prolonged dehydration, a stimulus for the release of histamine from its immune system side of activity will produce a greater quantity of its release into the tissues. At the same time, antibody production and efficiency, which have already been suppressed because of dehydration, will be inadequate to deal with foreign agents such as pollen and other antigens. The enormity of this problem becomes apparent during the pollen season when the eyes get invaded with these foreign agents. The tear-producing glands need to wash the offending pollen away from the delicate membrane of the eye—the conjunctiva—since antibodies are not adequately available to neutralize the pollen. This is the reason why histamine activity for secretion of water onto the delicate membranes covering the eyes and the nasal passages becomes exaggerated. It is a naturally installed need-driven response. "Water wash" is the only way of getting rid of the offending pollen types that are not neutralized by antibodies. This is how allergy to pollen occurs.

If you were to ask me: "Do you mean to say I can prevent asthma and allergies by drinking more water?" my answer would be yes, yes, and yes again. You can do it naturally, with no medication and at no cost. Water will do it because of the primary role of histamine in water regulation and drought management of the body.

It is now clear that chronic dehydration *is* the primary cause of allergies and asthma in the human body. Increased water intake—on a habit-forming, regular basis—should become the treatment of choice. In those who have attacks of asthma or allergic reactions to different pollens or foods, strict attention to adequate daily water intake, with the addition of some salt, should become a preventive measure. People who suffer from allergies and asthma will also have other indicators of dehydration. They will definitely develop other very serious health problems if they do not take their bodies' need for regular intake of water seriously. If you have any doubts about this information, read Andrew Bauman's letter, which follows.

If you suffer from allergies and asthma, you must begin by drinking water on a regular basis. You should stop taking caffeine and alcohol until your condition becomes normal. Those with normal heart and kidney functions should begin drinking two glasses of water a half hour before each meal, and one glass of water two and a half hours after the meal. When you increase your water intake, you also need to increase your salt intake to make up for the salt lost during increased urine production. Read more about salt in chapter 13.

Andrew Bauman suffered from different aspects of dehydration that emerged one after another, until he was told nothing could be done for him. His doctor advised him to put his affairs in order before his anticipated early death. Fortunately for him, he discovered the medicinal effects of water and is still alive. He has reversed the variety of problems produced by dehydration, save one condition that is gradually improving. Mr. Bauman's case history highlights the serious implications of allergies during childhood, which can lead to the development of serious diseases later in life if steps are not taken to hydrate the body adequately. For more information on asthma and allergies, and to read an abundance of testimonials from people who got rid of their problems, refer to my book *ABC of Asthma, Allergies and Lupus*.

November 13, 1998

Dear Dr. Batmanghelidj:

My name is Andrew J. Bauman IV, and I am 42 years young, yet at age 34 I felt and looked like I was at least 44! Most of my life has been spent battling illness and disease, whereas now I celebrate each moment of each day with a renewed vigor and vitality. I used to be chronically dehydrated and now I know better.

I was born on October 29, 1956, in Taylor, Pennsylvania. My parents lovingly cared for me—including having me vaccinated. I was reared on infant formula and later cereal, juices, and a small amount of water when I would cry from colic. After my first polio vaccine, I became mysteriously paralyzed from the waist down. Specialists were puzzled yet diagnosed "aborted polio." It left as suddenly as it appeared. When I received a booster dose of the vaccine at around age 5 in first grade, the paralysis returned. Months of hospitalization and bed rest resulted in my gaining weight. I mostly ate my meals and had visitors, drank soda and some water now and then—and once again the paralyzation disappeared.

When I began third grade—around eight years old—my allergic afflictions and symptoms had begun. I had problems with frequent dry coughs. I began experiencing some difficulties with breathing, itchy and watery eyes, and fatigue when I was around fresh-cut lawns from springtime until autumn. When I was a junior in high school, I experienced blackouts from allergies. Sometime around 1979, I saw a specialist who did testing and diagnosed me with allergies and asthma. I was treated with allergy shots and inhalers. The treatments just seemed to make things worse. My lips were always dry and cracked. At that time of my life I was drinking about 2 to 4 cups of coffee per day along with a few glasses of soda and some tea and alcohol.

I would have an occasional glass of water during the day. The allergies and asthma stayed with me until 1996 when my water intake was up to about two to three quarts a day. I no longer struggle with allergies or asthma.

My problems with diabetes began at age 14. I was diagnosed as an insulin-dependent or "juvenile diabetic." It was then that I began drinking diet beverages, including those with caffeine. My water intake at that time was still only around 2 to 4 glasses a day and I was drinking tea and started drinking coffee. The diabetes resulted in many hospitalizations over the years. By the mid-1980s I had problems with diabetic neuropathy, which was causing my legs to swell. I was scheduled to have dye injected into my legs to perform a diagnostic scan after a Doppler radar study showed some apparent blockages in the veins in my legs. The dye injections caused my veins to burst, which made the swelling get worse. I was then diagnosed with "venous insufficiency." In 1994, I was told that my legs would probably have to be removed within a year or so.

While attempting to get on a diabetic insulin supply trial, the initial examination revealed that the retinas in my eyes had grown blood vessels that were bleeding (diabetic retinopathy). I began receiving a series of laser surgeries over the next 15 years to attempt to seal the leaky vessels and to attempt to prevent any new vessel growth. This reduced my peripheral and night vision. In 1992, I developed an enlarged yet benign prostate gland and my kidneys began showing signs of deterioration. In 1993, I began experiencing some potency difficulties. In 1994, I began seeing a natural or homeopathic physician who, besides treating me with alternative medicine, advised me to increase my water intake. My intake of insulin was around 95 units of insulin daily.

In 1976, many immune system problems began developing. I developed infectious mononucleosis. In 1979, during one of my then frequent hospital stays, I was diagnosed with "mono" again! The doctors insisted that I shouldn't have "mono" again and began consulting with specialists. I received an influenza vaccine and was discharged—only to be readmitted a day later with a fever of 106 degrees F. I was undergoing many tests, however nothing much was showing up at that time. After many tests for severe abdominal pain, I was told that I grew a second spleen that was attached to my spleen and that the second one was also functioning. That year I was visiting someone and drank unpasteurized milk and ended up in the hospital again with a bacterial infection of the intestinal tract. "Brucellosis and Proteus OX-19" was the diagnosis and I was on yet more antibiotics.

During 1980 or 1981, I developed another case of "mono" and was admitted to the hospital again; diabetic control problems were a constant battle for me. An infectious disease specialist discovered that a number of special antibodies against foreign agents were also affected, which the doctors suggested were related to the problems with my allergies and asthma, as well as my frequent infections.

The 1980s were filled with many hospitalizations, illnesses, job losses, and stress-related problems. It was then that I was diagnosed with allergies to penicillin and tetracycline, began developing hypertension, was diagnosed with chronic fatigue syndrome, lymphoid hyperplasia (overstressed immune system), arthritis, bursitis, fibromyalgia, acid reflux problems, and bowel problems. I also developed a benign tumor on the left flank of my back. I developed a nodule on my thyroid area and was diagnosed with lead, cadmium, and aluminum poisoning, which were also found in a landfill I lived near. I was overweight and developed sleep apnea. Tests showed that I stopped breathing over 300 times in a six-hour period and had "narcolepsy." I could fall asleep in a short period of time. I had surgery to attempt to correct the sleep apnea, and I wore a tracheostomy tube in my neck to help me breathe at night, and slept with a breathing machine to keep my airway open. During the '80s I still only drank a few glasses of water daily, yet consumed large amounts of coffee, saccharine, and eventually NutraSweet. In 1987, I was declared "disabled."

In 1992, at 36 years old, I looked and felt like I was in my late forties and felt worse than I looked. I began using natural supplements with vitamins, herbs, and other natural medical techniques. The natural doctor's advice was to increase my water consumption and decrease my caffeine intake as well. I had lost the feeling in my feet, was always tired and achy, depressed, and had little hope.

I began to drink more water and reduced my caf-

*feine intake somewhat, and by 1995 I began to feel
and look much better. Yet I was still only consuming
a quart to a quart and a half daily, and not flushing
all the caffeine out of my system, nor was I using sea
salt.*

*In September of 1995, the lump on my left flank
turned red, began itching and enlarging. My family
physician removed it and sent it away for study. In
October, I was diagnosed with cutaneous B cell lymphoma. Twenty-six new tumors had grown on my
back where there was one, and I was sent to a major
hospital where I was told that lymphatic cancer on
the skin surface was rare and that not much research
was done yet on it. I went for a gallium scan and it
revealed that my entire body surface glowed positive
for cancer cells. The flank of my back was brighter
white or "hyperpositive," as was the middle of my
chest where two melanomas were previously
removed. I was advised to receive localized radiation,
and "as tumors appeared we would radiate them,
too," or I could travel to Philadelphia and have my
entire body surface radiated. They began to radiate
my back, which began giving me third-degree burns.
I refused total body radiation and, midway through
my radiation, my homeopathic physician began using
a natural cleansing therapy. The cancer specialist
had advised me to try anything and to "pull out all
the stops" as well as "to get my affairs in order." I
increased my water consumption and took supplements and natural treatments.*

*In November of 1995, while traveling in search
of an answer, I was introduced to a man who*

exposed me to your Water Cure program and advised me to stick to it very seriously to get cured. I now began to seriously increase my water intake, but was still leery of increasing salt intake due to the traditional medical contraindications for its perceived high blood pressure problems. Later I learned of the error of that thinking and began to increase my salt intake, too. In March of 1996, I went for another gallium scan, which revealed that there was not a single sign of cancer glowing positive on my entire body. Doctors thought there was an error in the gallium scan, but my homeopath and I knew that I was healing. Drinking more water, reducing caffeine, a change in dietary habits, natural medicine, and faith had brought me home.

Since then, I've been constantly improving in my health. I no longer have two spleens, but one that is normal in size and function. Now I lick sea salt off my palm in the morning before my first glass of water and use salt liberally. I drink about 1.5 gallons of water a day and take some supplements as well as eating a lot of whole grains, and fresh fruits and vegetables. My waist used to be a size 43 and now is a size 36. I weighed 249 pounds; now I weigh 210 and have solid muscle mass. My complexion and appearance are those of a man in his early thirties and my potency of a man in his twenties. My ankles are no longer swollen and new pulses, yes, new pulses, have developed where once they were dead. I no longer take any medications for all those problems, whereas I used to be on at least 15 prescriptions at a time. My insulin needs are down from 95 units a day to 35–45 units a day. I no longer suffer with "chronic infections" or fatigue—I sleep 6–8 hours a day instead of 12–14. It is rare for me to take an antibiotic, whereas I seemed to be constantly taking them before. I don't have allergies or asthma or gastroporesis (acid reflux) anymore. I no longer suffer from arthritis, bursitis, or bowel problems. At the time of my last stress test, my doctor, who is younger than I am, told me that I was in better shape than he was. The high blood pressure is constantly improving. No more thyroid nodule, I sleep better, and no more heavy metal toxicity. I have a new lease on life.

My prayers have been answered. God led me to a natural way to heal my body, my mind, and my spirit. I am living a new life now with a balance of water, salt, minerals, supplements, good nutrition, and continued improvements in my quality of life. I am truly blessed.

Sincerely,

Andrew J. Bauman IV

Michael P. is in his fifties. He suffered from allergies and eventually asthma since childhood. Later in life he became overweight and developed high blood pressure. His allergies were so bad that he had to pay attention to the daily pollen count before he could step out of the house. Several years ago he became aware of the curative properties of water in asthma and allergy. He started regulating his daily water intake and stopped drinking tea and coffee. When everyone in the office took coffee, he would drink hot water. Since then Michael has not had any asthma attacks. His allergy has become much less troublesome, almost to the point of being nonexistent. He no longer bothers with the pollen count. He has been free of allergy and asthma attacks since he started regulating his daily water intake. He considers himself cured of his health problems, including hypertension.

Question: Why is my doctor not aware of the information on water and asthma?

Answer: What I have shared with you so far is new knowledge. It has taken me more than twenty years of research and study to highlight this information. It is not yet common knowledge and is not yet taught at medical schools. Doctors recommend "fluid" intake and assume that any fluid you take will act like water. This is what doctors have been taught at medical school. They are not well informed about the intricate functions of water in the human body and do not yet understand chronic dehydration. They do not realize that not all fluids are suited to the normal physiological functions of the human body.

Furthermore, fluids that contain caffeine and alcohol dehydrate us and cannot replace the water needs of the human body. Caffeine and alcohol force the kidneys to flush some of the water reserves of the body.

Nathaniel C. is a young man in his twenties. He suffered from asthma since childhood. On several occasions, he developed attacks that needed immediate attention at the emergency department of the nearest hospital. One of these attacks was so severe that he needed to be hospitalized. Consequently, in constant fear of a repeat of these attacks, his inhaler was always with him and used frequently, possibly more often than prescribed. A good morning to him would mean a few puffs from his inhaler. He could not endure smoky rooms. He could not go through a business meeting without the support of his inhaler, nor could he exercise with the same abandon and pleasure as his friends. For Nathaniel, fear and the constant threat of another attack preoccupied his mind and punctuated the day's activity.

When he became aware of the topic of my research—chronic dehydration—he wanted to know if his asthma could be helped with water. He was surprised when I informed him that asthma was caused mainly by chronic dehydration. After adjusting his daily water intake and reducing his coffee intake, his breathing became more comfortable. He could go longer hours without needing his puffs of medication. He was able to reduce and eventually do away with his inhaler. He has been virtually free of his asthma and its associated fears for the past few years.

J. R., a physician, had developed adult-onset allergies and asthma when he was in college. At times he would get such severe attacks that he would need hospitalization for his suffocation and shocked state. He was allergic to cats more severely than other things.

He would never step into a house where there was a cat. Before accepting an invitation, he would ask if they kept a cat. Such was the state of his body sensitivity to some allergens.

One day while he was talking to me on the telephone, I noticed his repeated dry and gasping coughs. This was how I learned about his asthma. I asked him to drink a glass of water and put a pinch of salt on his tongue. His words: "As you recall, I was having a coughing spell that interrupted my work and, as you directed, the putting of some granules of salt on my tongue not only calmed my coughing but took it away: My nurses commented on my not coughing some five minutes later." For the past seven years he has been free of asthma and allergies. He seems not to fear cats anymore. He visits friends who have cats in their homes. He now treats his asthmatic patients with water and some added salt intake.

Asthma, in my opinion, is not a disease; it is a crisis complication of water shortage in the body. Anytime asthmatics do not drink enough water, their predisposition to asthma attacks will come back. You cannot be lazy about drinking water and expect asthma to stay away. Many people who get well and think the problem is over get a rude shock when shortness of breath begins again once they slack off from the routine. We now know the cause of asthma—dehydration. If we can get this simple understanding of asthma into the minds of the American public, I believe we can easily *eradicate asthma* from the list of health concerns in this country, and the rest of the world, in less than five years.

Let me share with you a story that happened recently. I was discussing the various complications of dehydration during an interview on a popular local radio show. A lady called to thank a friend of mine for having disseminated information about asthma and dehydration in that part of the world.

The listener then told me she has two small children in her family, three and four years old. Two winters ago both youngsters suffered from severe asthma, which caused their family great concern. At the beginning of last year she increased their water intake. The result: These children no longer suffer from asthma—not even one episode the whole of last winter. She also told us how her husband's insulin-dependent diabetes has started improving since he has increased his water intake. He now needs much less insulin to manage his daily life. Her daughter also suffered from severe back pain and was diagnosed with lumbar disc degeneration and atrophy. She, too, went on The Water Cure and is now pain-free.

From one person in this family taking the information on chronic dehydration seriously and acting on The Water Cure recommendations, four of her family members are no longer in serious danger from the complications of dehydration. An important aspect of their discovery about water is their freedom from medical ignorance that would have treated their health problems with chemical products or invasive procedures that would have drastically compromised their health and financial resources.

Increased food intake, when not accompanied by increased water intake, will also produce susceptibility to allergies. If you remember, food-laden, concentrated blood has to circulate through the lungs and further give up some of its water through evaporation. People with allergies and asthma should make it a habit to drink water before eating their food—at least a few minutes before beginning. At no time should they allow food intake to concentrate their body fluids to the extent that high levels of histamine generation become a permanent situation.

Question: What is wrong with waiting until you feel thirsty to drink water?

Answer: The body is already thirsty before we feel the thirst sensation. Dry mouth is not an accurate sign of water shortage in our body. There is a mechanism by which, even when we are comparatively dehydrated, saliva production is not affected. The reason is that we must be able to lubricate food during the process of chewing and swallowing. The misconception about dry mouth as an accurate indicator of body-water shortage has steered the trends in medical research off course, so that, even today, it is not generally known at what stage the body is thirsty and becoming pathologically dehydrated. It is not fully appreciated what devastating damage is caused by a slowly establishing dehydration in the body.

If children are not able to regulate their water intake properly, histamine activity in the lungs may become a dominant trend. One of the consequences of overactivity of histamine in the lungs may be the occurrence of an inflammatory process at a time when the development of lung tissue has to keep up with the physical growth of the body. Excessive fibrous tissue formation and the creation of cysts where alveoli have to be formed may be the consequence of dehydration in children who are growing. It seems that cystic fibrosis of the lungs may not be an entirely genetic disorder, but may have dehydration as a common basic problem to both the DNA assembly system and lung tissue formation. Dehydration is also responsible for the production of excess thick mucus in the bronchioles—a problem in cystic fibrosis of the lungs. Water and salt should help loosen the mucus.

Children need water for cell growth. During growth, 75 percent of the cell volume has to be filled with water. This is the reason why children develop asthma and allergies during the growing phase of their physical development.

As we grow older, we lose our thirst sensation and do not recognize that our body is thirsty. Chronic dehydration in the elderly can cause heart and kidney damage, coupled with shortness of breath. At this stage, the shortness of breath is called cardiac asthma. Those with heart problems and kidney disease should increase their water intake slowly and, if possible, under the supervision of their physicians. They need to make sure their urine production increases with the additional water. If within two full days there is no indication of more urine being produced, a physician should be consulted. The color of urine in a dehydrated person (not taking vitamins that could color the urine) will be dark yellow to orange. *In a better-hydrated person, the urine is lighter in color.*

Children and adults who get asthma attacks with exercise and strenuous effort should always remember to drink water before they begin exercising and to stop drinking caffeine-containing sodas. They should reduce their orange juice intake (if more than two glasses). Because of its high potassium content, too much orange juice can predispose a person to asthma attacks. The water needs of the body cannot be fully replaced by juices or even milk.

On no account should you abruptly cut off the use of your medications. You should begin by taking more water with your medications, until your need for medication decreases. Keep the doctor in charge of your treatment informed. You will then be able to work with your doctor to gradually reduce the use of the normally prescribed inhalant or antihistamine medications until you no longer need them. In obstinate and truly drug-dependent cases of asthma and allergies, increased water intake will improve the patient's response to the medications being prescribed until the body gets back to its normal rhythm.

The choice of water should not become a limiting factor to drinking it. So long as tap water contains no lead, mercury, pesticides, insecticides, or other dangerous chemicals or bacteria, it should become your fluid of choice. It is available to you everywhere you go. You should not worry about its hardness. Any calcium that is dissolved in water may even serve a useful purpose, as it might help your body's need for calcium.

If the smell of chlorine is too much, fill an open-top jug and leave it exposed to air. The chlorine will evaporate in less than a half hour, and the water will be sweet and ready to drink.

It is becoming fashionable to advocate drinking distilled water. This claim may prove to be based on the commercial aims of its manufacturers. I have found no reason to drink distilled water over regular tap water that does not contain toxic substances. If you are unsure of your local water, it would be a good idea to install a solid carbon filter on your kitchen faucet.

With increased water intake, which will cause increased urine production, there may be an associated loss of salt, as well as other minerals and water-soluble vitamins. Supplementing your daily vitamin intake is necessary. If you develop cramps, you should assume that the salt in your diet is not sufficient for your body's needs. You should add salt to your diet—as long as you stick to taking more water. In asthma and allergy sufferers, salt intake becomes a vital part of the treatment. Salt unplugs the thick mucus secretions in the lungs and stops the overflow of nasal secretion, *when water is plentiful*. Salt breaks up mucus, rendering it watery and stringy, and suitable for expulsion with the flow of sputum, when water is also available.

I recommend to asthmatics who are about to get an attack, or are in the middle of an asthma attack, to drink two or three glasses of water, and then put a pinch of salt on their tongue. Water and salt will tell the brain that the missing components in a dehydrated body—in asthmatics in particular—have entered the system. The brain will immediately instruct the bronchioles to relax, and breathing will become much easier. When the salt reaches the lungs, salt pumps secrete it in the bronchioles to loosen the mucus plugs and prepare them to be carried away— *only when water is available*. Too much salt and *not enough water* may do the opposite. It might cause constriction of the bronchioles.

This is why phlegm always tastes salty. Salt is essential to keep the airways of the body clear—including the nasal passageways when you have a cold. Salt also unplugs mucus in the nose and the sinuses and stops runny nose in allergic reactions.

BLOOD PRESSURE AND DEHYDRATION

The measurable force that rushes blood through the arterial system of the body is called blood pressure. This force has two components. The diastolic component is the constant basic force in the arteries that keeps the blood vessels full and under a constant basic pressure. It is the lowest reading on the measuring instruments. The normally accepted figure for this reading is between 60 and 90. The systolic component of blood pressure is the sharp rise in force inside the arteries, produced by the contraction of the left side of the heart when it forces the volume of blood in its ventricle into an already filled and under-pressure arterial system. The normal range is between 90 and 130. In other words, the accepted normal blood pressure—systolic over diastolic—is from 90 over 60 to 130 over 90.

The difference in the two readings is significant. It

means that the blood is being stirred by the rush of new blood in the arteries, which prevents blood's heavier constituents from sedimenting in the stagnant areas; it means an added pressure that will squirt some clear serum through the tiny holes in the capillaries and into the filtration areas in the kidneys for cleansing of the blood. The significance of the diastolic pressure is in its effect of filling all the blood vessels of the body so none remains empty.

The problem of blood circulation becomes apparent if the diastolic pressure rises well above or falls well below the normal range. If it rises above the range, it means the heart has much more pressure to work against when forcing blood into the circulation. For a short period of time, it is not a big deal. But given sixty to eighty beats a minute, day in and day out, you will have one very tired heart, as well as overshocked blood vessels that have to become thick and inelastic to withstand the repeated onslaught. Diastolic pressure well below normal affects circulation, especially to the brain. Not enough pressure in the arteries that go to the brain means less oxygen reaching the vital brain centers. The result: feeling faint and not fully focused. With low blood pressure, you can actually faint if you stand up suddenly. How do these complications arise? *Dehydration!*

High Blood Pressure

Roughly sixty million Americans suffer from hypertension or high blood pressure. There may be more than one reason when blood pressure readings register an increase from what is considered normal. In my scientific opinion, the most common and frequent reason is a gradually establishing dehydration in the body. This type of hypertension is labeled "essential hypertension." A large number of people in this group receive some form of medication to deal with this dehydration signal of the body. Until they learn about the relationship of this condition to their insufficient water intake, or a wrong choice of fluid intake, they will have to continue taking pharmaceutical products for the rest of their shortened lives.

The paradigm shift offers us a new perspective on high blood pressure—the form we call essential hypertension. It tells us that a gradual rise in blood pressure is an indicator of a gradually establishing shortage of water in the body. The blood vessels of the body have been designed to cope with repeated fluctuations in their blood volume and the circulation requirements of the tissues they supply. They have tiny holes or lumen that open and close to adapt to the amount of blood inside them. In water loss from the body—rather, lack of sufficient water intake—66 percent of the deficit is reflected in the volume of water held in some cells of the body (plumlike cells begin to become prunelike); 26 percent is reflected in the fluid environment outside the cells; and only 8 percent of the deficit is imposed on the volume held in blood circulation. The circulatory system adapts to its 8 percent loss by shrinking in capacity. Initially, peripheral capillaries close down, and eventually the larger vessels tighten their walls to keep the blood vessels full.

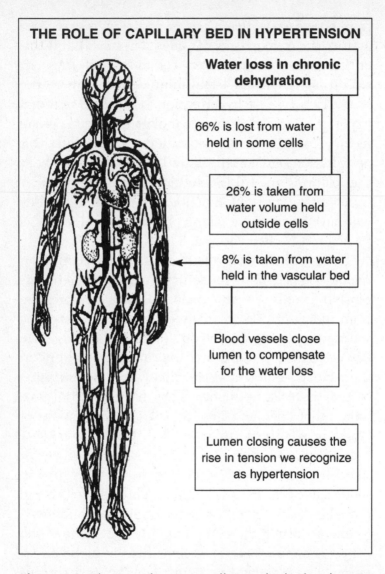

THE ROLE OF CAPILLARY BED IN HYPERTENSION

Water loss in chronic dehydration

66% is lost from water held in some cells

26% is taken from water volume held outside cells

8% is taken from water held in the vascular bed

Blood vessels close lumen to compensate for the water loss

Lumen closing causes the rise in tension we recognize as hypertension

Figure 7.1: The vascular system all over the body adapts to blood volume loss by selective closing of the lumen. One major cause for blood volume loss is the loss of body water or its undersupply through the loss of thirst sensation.

This tightening leads to a measurable rise in tension in the arteries. This is called hypertension. If the blood vessels did not tighten on the void, gases would separate from the blood and fill the space, causing gas locks. This vascular adaptation to the amount of water the vascular system carries is a most advanced design within the principle of hydraulics that the blood circulation of the body is modeled on.

Injection Pressure for the Filter Systems

Another major reason for the tightening of the vessels is the need to squeeze the blood volume in the arterial system so that water can be filtered and injected into some vitally important cells in the body, such as the brain cells. The tightening of the blood vessel walls provides the force necessary to operate a reverse osmosis system in the human body—a crisis-management program to keep important cells alive. Water is pushed into selected cells of the body through tiny "showerheads"—cluster perforations in the cell membrane. The difference between the two readings of blood pressure is the range of force needed to deliver water under normal circumstances into some vital cells of the body. As the body becomes more and more dehydrated, the amount of pressure needed to filter and inject water into vital cells increases. The less water there is in the body, the more pressure is needed to hydrate vital cells.

The mechanism is simple. When confronting stressful circumstances, and in dehydration that is becoming gradually established, histamine is released. Histamine activates the production of vasopressin (an antidiuretic hormone). Certain cells of the body have receiving points that are sensitive to vasopressin. As soon as the hormone sits on the sensitive point, a hollow showerhead type of opening with minute holes in its base is created in the cell membrane. Serum fills the space, and its water content filters through the holes, which are large enough for the passage of only one water molecule at a time. Vasopressin, as its name implies, also produces the tightening of the vessels around it. This tightening of vessels translates into a squeeze that pushes the serum and its water through the holes in the blood vessel—a necessary act if some of this water is to be pushed back into the cells.

Renin-Angiotensin System

Another water-regulatory system that is associated with dehydration and histamine production is the brain's renin-angiotensin (RA) system. RA production is a component of the thirst sensation and increased water intake. It also produces some tightening of the blood vessels and has been recognized as a dominant factor in the production of hypertension. The RA system eventually becomes prominent in the kidneys, which have to concentrate urine and save water while producing urine. The kidneys recognize water shortage and activate their resident RA system so that more water is called in for urine production. The RA system eventually stimulates a drive for salt

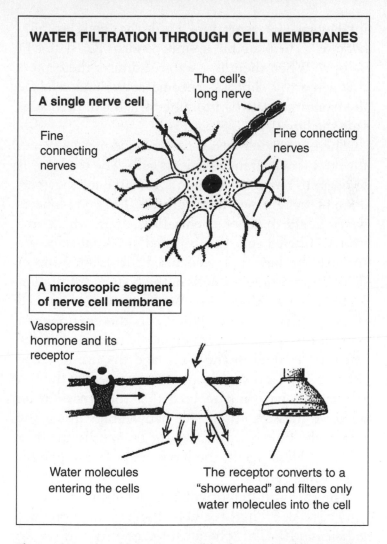

WATER FILTRATION THROUGH CELL MEMBRANES

The cell's long nerve

A single nerve cell

Fine connecting nerves

Fine connecting nerves

A microscopic segment of nerve cell membrane

Vasopressin hormone and its receptor

Water molecules entering the cells

The receptor converts to a "showerhead" and filters only water molecules into the cell

Figure 7.2: The schematic model of a nerve cell, its membrane wall, and the vasopressin receptor that becomes transformed into a type of "showerhead" that lets only water through its very small perforations. This is part of the mechanism of reverse osmosis that the body employs to deliver filtered water into vital cells.

intake and its retention until the body is fully hydrated. The brain has an independent RA system of its own. When there is a water shortage, the centers that sense this shortage become active and produce the neurotransmitter histamine, which will then activate the brain's RA system.

There is a simultaneous rise in blood pressure when the body is dehydrated inside its cells. The tendency is to begin to retain salt, which is essential for the operation of the reverse osmosis process. The body collects water in the form of edema fluid, from which free water is filtered and then injected into vital cells. We in medicine have not recognized the relationship of dehydration inside the cells of the body to the physiological role of RA system. We have only recognized the expansion of water volume in the environment outside the cells. We automatically assume that the retention of fluid in the body, and the rise in blood pressure, are pathological processes caused by the RA system. We have not realized that the process is an adaptive measure to correct dehydration inside the vital cells of the body, such as the brain cells, the liver cells, the kidney cells, the lungs, and other important organs and glands.

The chemical steps involve angiotensin-converting enzymes (ACE). In three steps, these enzymes produce *angiotensin III*. This chemical forces a strict drive for retention of salt in the body. Extra salt will retain extra water in the tissues. *The only things that turn off this salt-retaining-drive mechanism are adequate water intake and some salt intake that balance the fluid content inside and outside the cells. The salt should be unrefined sea salt that contains other vital minerals that are needed to hold on to the water once it is injected or diffused inside the cells.*

When it is freely available, water diffuses quite rapidly through the cell membranes without needing to be forced. Its rate of diffusion through the cell membrane has been calculated to be 10^{-3} centimeters per second, which is fairly fast. This natural and fast diffusion process of water in the kidneys is the reason why water itself is a natural diuretic—far better than chemical diuretics or ACE inhibitors now used routinely. In fact, to give a person with essential hypertension diuretics is, in my opinion, a blatant disservice to the patient.

Water itself will increase urine production, and excess retained salt will gradually be passed in the urine. This is why water is a most effective decongestant and edema remover. When you drink water to dilute the blood, it will not be necessary to rely entirely on the process of reverse osmosis and the RA system to force water into vital cells—including the renal tissue that has to make concentrated urine and force the toxic waste out of the body. The body will not cause a collection of extra fluid in the tissues as a reservoir to filter and inject water into its vital cells as an emergency process. This is what essential hypertension is all about.

Because it is associated with aging, and seemed unavoidable in the past, the gradual rise in blood pressure has been labeled "essential hypertension," meaning it is an unavoidable outcome of living to a mature life. It was not recognized that a gradual loss of thirst perception as we grow older is responsible for the onset of chronic dehydration and subsequent hypertension.

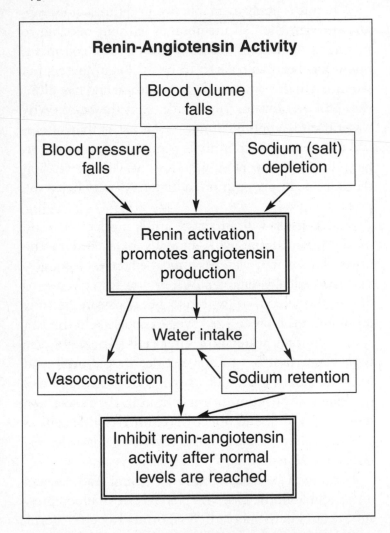

Figure 7.3: A model of physiological events that will either stimulate or inhibit renin-angiotensin production.

Naturally, an increase in daily water intake and sea salt that contains other minerals will correct this problem. The present way of dealing with hypertension is criminal. To give diuretics to a hypertensive who has adequate kidney function is absurd. The body is trying to retain its water by storing salt, and we say to the design of nature in us: "No, you do not understand, you must take diuretics and get rid of water." By giving diuretics and reducing the water content of the body, we reduce the efficiency of the reverse osmosis system that is delivering water to the brain and other important cells in the body. Water by itself is the best natural diuretic. It should be remembered that complications associated with hypertension, including coronary thrombosis and repeated strokes, are, in effect, caused by persistent dehydration. Remember: Chronic dehydration kills prematurely and painfully. The use of diuretics assists in the process.

Truck driver Jim Bolen, whose letter follows, is an extremely interesting person. He was trained as a pilot and worked with one of the airlines. Because of very high blood pressure he was grounded, unable to fly any longer. This is when he discovered The Water Cure and was able to lower his blood pressure with ease and without any of the usual chemicals that are prescribed for this condition. By nature, he is very inquisitive and curious to learn. He has a sharp memory for detail. He has taken to heart the information on the role of water and its curative properties and is determined to enlighten and help others.

Bolen is now a traveling missionary for The Water Cure. He drives a truck the length and the breadth of the country. He talks to other drivers at truck stops or through their system of radio communication. He gets them to drink water when they are tired and feel sleepy at the wheel. He gets them to give up their caffeine-containing coffee and sodas and drink water instead. He tells them about the importance of adequate salt intake in proportion to the amount of water they need. Every month, he buys several hundred dollars' worth of books and tapes and gives them to the people who need the information to improve their health. He stops at churches and parishes on his way. He talks to priests on his delivery routes and gives them books and videotapes to share with their parishioners. He has helped thousands of people learn about the importance of water in their lives.

TO: *Dr. Batman*

FROM: *Jim Bolen*

I discovered the importance of water and salt to the human body in June of 1997 when I failed a medical for renewing my commercial flying license My pressure at rest was 230/110. I was grounded and told to see my personal physician. He told me I needed blood pressure medication, but I decided I was not going on any medication yet.

I left upset, in denial. My blood pressure had always been 120/80. I got a second opinion weeks later after trying garlic, herbs, vitamins, exercise, meditation, and found it still a solid 180/100. He told me if I didn't go on medication, my heart would enlarge and I would have a heart attack or stroke down the road.

I went home, depressed. I didn't want to accept old age at 54. I was telling a friend about my situation when a retired chiropractor told me about your book (Your Body's Many Cries for Water). He loaned me his book and told me to stop all caffeine for a week, drink ten glasses of water, and add ½ tsp of salt to my diet.

I looked at him like he was crazy. I had been on a salt-free diet for years. Thank God for your book, Dr. Batmanghelidj, and Dr. Lee Hobson for his time and generosity.

My blood pressure is now 117/75. I'm taking no medication at all and I have unlimited energy at 58 years old. No more headache or lower back pain; sinuses are clear and no constipation.

Thankfully,

Jim Bolen
Indio, CA

I could write much more about blood pressure. Suffice it to say, "essential hypertension" is an indicator of an establishing chronic dehydration. Correct the established dehydration in your body with an adjustment to daily water intake and adequate intake of minerals to replace those lost through increased urination, and the adaptive need to raise the blood pressure from its normal levels will not arise. It is as simple as that. Dehydration is by far the most frequent constant stressor in the human body that raises blood pressure—in at least sixty million Americans. However, there may arise occasions when other silent stressors may bring about the same chemical driving forces that ultimately raise blood pressure. These occasions are few and far between and need exhaustive investigation to pinpoint the problem. We need to exclude dehydration as the primary cause of the rise in blood pressure first, before embarking on other approaches.

Salt and Hypertension

Recent articles in scientific journals are also questioning the view that salt is bad for those with hypertension. Dr. H. Alderman of Albert Einstein College of Medicine and associates, in their 1995 article in the *Journal of Hypertension,* have shown that people on restrictively low-salt diets are more likely to die from heart attacks or strokes than those who use salt liberally. In a 1997 article in the *American Journal of Clinical Nutrition,* Dr. David McCurron of the Department of Nephrology at Oregon Health Science University, Portland, found that with adequate daily intake of potassium, calcium, and magnesium, not only will salt not raise blood pressure, it might actually lower it. This article confirms my view that the water volume inside and outside the cells of the body needs to be in balance. Remember that salt regulates the water levels outside the cells. Potassium, magnesium, and calcium are the vital minerals that balance the water volume inside the cells.

Additional information you need to remember is that five elements—water, salt, potassium, magnesium, and caicium—are involved in energy regulation inside the cells. *Water drives the sodium potassium pump protein and manufactures hydroelectricity.* This hydroelectricity is used for immediate needs, and the excess of it is converted to usable stored energy for emergency use. Calcium is bonded to other calcium in bones and in the endoplasmic reticulum inside the cells. Each bonded calcium atom traps one unit of energy that can be reused if necessary. Magnesium traps many units of energy in the form of magnesium ATP.

As you can see, the mystery of essential hypertension is solved. To avoid the problem, you need to take an adequate amount of water daily so that the urine is light in color. Your diet should include no less than 3 to 4 grams of salt, about 1 gram of calcium, 400 to 800 milligrams of magnesium (although this amount of magnesium is more than the official dietary reference values, most people are severely magnesium-deficient and need to correct the deficiency), and about 2,000 to 4,000 milligrams of potassium. It is easy to get the potassium in high-potassium foods such as raisins, potatoes, avocados, lima and all the other beans, peas, tomatoes, cauliflower, bananas, bread, oranges, grapefruits, dried apricots, milk, eggs, and cheese. Practically everything you eat has some potassium content. You need to eat foods and fruits with higher potassium content.

If you do not eat kelp, wheat bran, wheat germ, almonds, and other nuts that have very high magnesium content, or green leafy vegetables in which magnesium is a component of chlorophyll, you should take magnesium supplements every day. As for calcium, in order of their calcium content, kelp, cheese, sesame seeds, bean curd, molasses, pulses—lentils, different beans—figs, almonds, spring greens, watercress, parsley, plain yogurt, shrimp, broccoli, milk, cottage cheese, and olives will provide the calcium needs of the body. People on weight-loss programs, or those who do not have access to a balanced diet, should take these minerals in the form of supplements.

Iodine is a very important element for the regulation of the fluid content of the body. Iodine is essential for the thyroid gland to manufacture thyroxin, its primary hormone. It seems that thyroxin is the element that stimulates the cells to manufacture all the pump proteins that regulate the sodium, potassium, and other mineral balances outside and inside the cells, and that generate energy in the process. With the movement of sodium and potassium across the cell membrane, not only will water also move to balance the osmotic pressure in and out of the cell, but the other mineral-transferring pumps will take their cue and regulate the magnesium, potassium, and calcium levels of the cell interior as well.

Before salt was iodized, many people suffered from iodine deficiency and lumpy thyroid gland enlargement in their necks, known as thyroid goiter. One of the major complications of iodine deficiency is the collection of hard-to-move and inelastic swelling and edema, known as myxedema. Other complications are dry skin, loss of hair and memory, tiredness, sleepiness, and loss of muscle tissue. As you can see, iodine is vital for good health and good fluid balance.

Much to my regret, I discovered that unrefined sea salt does not have enough iodine. Thinking that sea salt has many important trace elements, I switched to using only sea salt and was not diligent in taking foods and multivitamins that would provide my body with the iodine it needs. My second mistake was that being so busy with sharing my medical breakthrough on water metabolism of the body with people that I was not alert to my own health problems. I developed all the early stages of iodine deficiency, but no goiter in my neck. However, I developed an uncomfortable feeling in my chest and also shortness of breath.

A high-resolution CT scan of my chest revealed a massive thyroid goiter in my chest that was pressing on my trachea, to the point of deforming it. This was three months ago. I adjusted my iodine intake in the form of dried kelp or as part of the composition of the one-a-day multivitamin that I now take religiously. As a result, my breathing problem has cleared, my edema has cleared, I am no longer lethargic, and my energy level has increased; my sleep has normalized; my blood pressure is back to the normal range. I now feel much healthier and more confident and have lost fifteen pounds of the swelling that I had amassed. All these improvements have been made possible because of the vital role of simple iodine in the physiology of the body and adjustment to my intake of vital minerals mentioned above. You see, even doctors get sick, and that is how we learn. A word of caution: Do not overdo iodine intake. It could cause other problems.

DIABETES

Diabetes seems to be the end result of water deficiency in the brain, to the point that the brain's neurotransmitter systems, particularly the system that is regulated by the neurotransmitter serotonin, are affected. It is within the automatic design of the brain to peg up the glucose threshold so that it can maintain its own volume and energy requirements when there is a water shortage in the body. When there is a gradually establishing chronic dehydration in the body, the brain has to depend more on glucose as a source of energy. The brain needs more glucose for its energy value and its metabolic conversion to water. Under the urgent circumstances produced by stress, up to 85 percent of the supplemental energy requirement by the brain is provided by sugar alone. This is why stressed people resort to eating sweet food. While all the other cells need to be influenced by insulin to take up glucose through their cell walls, the brain does not depend on insulin to carry sugar across its cell membranes.

It seems to be in the natural design of the brain to steer the physiological mechanisms in the direction of higher glucose level in the body when there is persistent dehydration that would damage the brain more than it could recover from. The brain resuscitates itself in the same way that a doctor resuscitates a patient—with intravenous fluid containing sugar and salt. The main problem stems from one very important factor—the salt metabolism (both sodium and potassium) of the body also becomes negatively affected when there is water deficiency in the body. This condition should be treated with an increase in water intake and diet manipulation to provide the necessary minerals and amino acid balance for tissue repair—including brain tissue requirements.

It has been shown that the brain amino acid balance for tryptophan is affected in diabetic rats. There seems to be a much lower level of this amino acid in the brain when diabetes exists. Tryptophan in turn regulates the salt intake of the body. Salt is responsible for regulating water-volume content outside the cells of the body. When there is tryptophan deficiency in the body, there is also a total body-salt shortage. With lower salt retention as a result of tryptophan deficiency, the responsibility for holding water in the body and outside the cells falls onto the sugar content in the blood. To do its new job, and compensate for the lower salt, the sugar content rises. The way this happens is so simple it is almost unbelievable.

One of histamine's deputies, which becomes increasingly active in water-distribution systems, is prostaglandin E. This chemical inhibits the insulin-making cells in the pancreas, preventing them from making and secreting insulin. When insulin is not adequately secreted, the main body cells do not receive sufficient sugar and some amino acids. Potassium stays outside the cells, and the water that accompanies potassium does not enter the cells, either. In this way, the cells of the body are forced to forgo their right to water and some amino acids, and they gradually become damaged. This is how diabetes becomes the cause of many associated disease conditions.

Diabetes is a good example of next-generation

damage that is caused by dehydration. Whereas the onset of dehydration-induced diabetes is normally seen in the elderly and is often reversible, the more structurally serious and irreversible variety of the disease is seen in younger people. The juvenile variety of diabetes needs to be treated carefully before it becomes a totally irreversible type of diabetes and permanent structural damage takes place. Basically the cause is the same in children as in adults, except that in adults there is more "reserve in the system." In children, the process of physical growth strains the system much more quickly. Children are constantly dehydrated, and their amino acid pool is in a state of constant fluctuation.

At the moment, there seems to be total reliance on the belief that genetic dictation is what promotes the occurrence of diabetes, particularly in the young. One important fact to remember is that the DNA structure is held together by proteins that also obey the many dictates of water as their ultimate regulator. Water is the common factor for all protein functions in the body, including the DNA-manufacturing system. Accordingly, the associated genetic marker in diabetes may not be a dictating factor for disease production; rather, it may be the indicator of a deep-rooted, dehydration-caused damage that has also affected the DNA recording system—a passive outcome.

Pancreas: The Failed Organ in Diabetes

The pancreas, where insulin is made, is an organ that is directly involved in the regulation of the balance between the water compartments of the body. The water volume held inside each cell is regulated and held by the amount of potassium that is forced into the cell. Insulin is a very effective agent for forcing potassium (and amino acids) inside the cells. If potassium stays outside the cells and in circulation, at a certain threshold it can produce irregular heartbeats and, often, a sudden heart seizure and stopping of the heart's rhythmic contractions. In effect, therefore, insulin regulates water volume inside the cell. It manages this responsibility by pushing potassium and sugar into the cell that has insulin-sensitive gates of entry on its outer membrane.

The pancreas has another equally important responsibility. It has to collect water from some of its cells, mix it with manufactured bicarbonate and pancreatic enzymes, and secrete the mixture into the intestine to neutralize the acid that is poured into the intestine from the stomach and begin the next phase of digestion of food. The mixture is known as *watery bicarbonate solution*.

The Role of the Pancreas in Water Rationing

If water is in short supply, the watery bicarbonate solution that is secreted into the intestine cells may not be enough to neutralize all the acid that enters the intestine to begin the cycle of food digestion. Consequently, one or the other process has to be halted. Either the acid has to stop coming into the intestine, or water has to be delivered to the pancreas in a sufficient amount for the pancreas to perform at least one of its functions. A commensurate reduction of insulin secretion stops the entry of water and nutrients into the peripheral cells in the rest of the body that depend on the presence of insulin for their feeding process. By this process, more water will be available in the circulating blood to be delivered to the pancreas to make its watery bicarbonate solution. When the insulin-stimulated gates are not efficient in delivering water and raw materials into the cells, they begin to wither and die. This is the mechanism behind the degenerative process associated with diabetes.

In dyspeptic cases, acid will continue to build up in the stomach. The ring muscle between the stomach and the intestine will close the gap, and nothing will enter the intestine. The more the stomach contracts to push its load into the intestine, the tighter the ring will contract. Only a fraction of the load is let out. Over time, ulcerations in the ring area are produced. In this situation, the full acid load does not enter into the intestine, and less demand is placed on the pancreas for secretion of its watery bicarbonate solution.

In diabetes, the action of insulin in pushing water into the cells is stopped. This is done simply by a two-step process: The first step, a reversible one, is to prevent insulin secretion from the cells that manufacture it. This type of diabetes is called insulin-independent diabetes. The pancreas has the ability to secrete insulin. A second, and much more drastic, ruthless, and irreversible way, is to destroy the insulin-making cells. The process involves the destruction of their nuclei. Enough of their DNA/RNA system is dismembered to make them ineffective as insulin producers. This kind of diabetes is known as insulin-dependent or type I diabetes.

Insulin-Independent Diabetes

This form of diabetes is often reversible. When the insulin-secreting cells are temporarily inhibited by prostaglandin E, certain outside agents can override this and get insulin released. The knowledge of this process of insulin release has been used in devising a simpler treatment procedure than insulin injections. The agents that release insulin are given in tablet form, usually one tablet once a day.

These tablets are normally given to elderly diabetics and not to young ones. There are side effects to these tablets, including abnormalities in blood cell count and blood cell composition, jaundice, gastrointestinal symptoms, liver-function problems, and skin rashes. Hypoglycemic coma is also a complication of overdose of these tablets, often the result of forgetful repeat of medication. The use of these drugs is dangerous in liver disease and kidney-function irregularities or deficiency.

In insulin-independent diabetes, a regular daily adjustment of water intake to no less than two quarts, and some increased salt intake, is the best treatment. In this form of diabetes, when the body makes some insulin but does not release it because of the effect of prostaglandin E, water intake and adjustment of diet and minerals often will reverse the situation, and the need for higher blood sugar will subside.

Insulin-Dependent Diabetes

Diabetes can become permanently established when there is DNA/RNA damage. In this type of diabetes, the ability to manufacture insulin is lost. If prostaglandin E remains in general circulation long enough, it activates the hormone interleukin-6. This chemical works its way into the nucleus of insulin-producing cells and gradually dismembers the DNA/RNA scaffolding of the nucleus, decreasing its size and reducing its ability to function. Thus water deficiency, if uncorrected for a long time, can in many people cause damage—sometimes permanent—to their insulin-producing cells.

Subsequently, even more damage to the diabetic body can occur. Some organs begin to suffer and become useless. A leg can shrink and become gangrenous, if not amputated; cysts can form in the brain; eyes can become blind.

Diabetes in Children

In children, the process is the same, except it begins at a much earlier age until it becomes an "autoimmune" disease. That is to say, the insulin-producing cells are destroyed to avoid the need for constant control of their activity (see figure 7.4). The body of a child has much less water reserve than that of a grown person. It seems logical to assume that the gap between the inhibition of insulin release and the threshold of insulin cell destruction must also be less wide. Adding to this problem is the fact that a growing body is always dehydrated. Every cell in the soft tissues needs about 75 percent of its volume to be water to function within the norms of the human body.

When the body is growing under the influence of growth hormone, as well as other hormones, and the effect of histamine with its food- and water-supply regulation, a form of stress is constantly experienced. This stimulates the thirst sensation, and the body will demand water. Plain water should be given, although some parents force their own habits of drinking sodas, tea, or juices on their children.

Nothing—but nothing—can substitute for water to satisfy the water needs of the body. It is true that other drinks contain some water, but they do not affect the body in the same way as water itself. The vitamins contained in fresh fruit juices are essential for the body. Still, too much of any juice—particularly orange and grapefruit juice—can be harmful. Juices can increase the acidity of the intestine and then the body. Their high potassium content can drastically increase the activation and presence of histamine. This will signal undue stress to the body, and a crisis water-rationing state will develop.

The physical growth of the body of a child is an adaptive response to the stresses and demands placed on it. It grows as a result of this stress, and histamine's activities are an essential part of the process.

CONSTIPATION AND ITS COMPLICATIONS

The intestinal tract uses much water to break down solid foods. It has to liquefy the dissolvable components of solid foods to extract their essential elements. Whatever can be dissolved is then absorbed into the blood circulation and transferred to the liver for processing. The refuse that cannot be further broken down is then passed on through the various segments of the gut and gradually compacted for elimination.

Depending on the adequate availability of free water in the body, the refuse will carry with it some of the water that was used to liquefy the food. What water it can carry with it will act as a lubricant to help the refuse move through the large intestine. The last segments of the small intestine and most of the large intestine are under the direction of the water regulators to reabsorb as much of the water in the refuse as might be needed by the other parts of the body. The more the body is in need of water, the more there is a determined effort to reabsorb the water that is available in the intestine. This process puts a drastic squeeze on the refuse to separate its water content and make it available for reabsorption by the mucosa or lining membranes of the large intestine.

The more the body is dehydrated, the slower the motility of the lower intestines in order to allow time for reabsorption of the water content of the refuse. This process of preventing water loss is another of the body's water-preservation mechanisms. One part of the body where water loss is prevented in times of drought management is in the large intestine, through adjustment of the consistency and the rate of flow of the excrements. When the passage of refuse from the large intestine is slowed down, the mucosa absorb the water, and the feces become hard and not fluid enough to flow. The act of expulsion of solid feces becomes difficult. To prevent this process from taking place, added intake of water and some fibers that hold the water better seems to be the only natural solution to constipation. Remember that hemorrhoids, diverticulitis, and polyp formation are common occurrences with chronic constipation. Chronic dehydration and its consequential constipation are primers for cancer formation in the large intestine and the rectum.

Reabsorption of water in the digestive tract also involves the regulating valve between the last part of the small intestine and the first part of the large intestine, known as the ileocecal valve. The valve shuts down and allows the small intestine time to get as much water as possible out of the as-yet-unformed refuse. At certain levels of dehydration, the closing of the valve may become too forceful and may cause spasm. This spasm will translate into pain in the lower right side of the abdomen. This pain can be mistaken for a possible inflammation of the appendix, which is served by the same sensory nerves. In women, this same pain could be misdiagnosed as either ovarian pain or uterine pain, which can cause anxiety and result in expensive, complicated investigations. Let me give you an example.

Joy is one of my assistants at Global Health Solutions. For the past few months, she was suffering from an uncomfortable pain in the area of her appendix—

the lower right side of her abdomen. She was advised by her doctor to have a laparoscopy to see what was causing her pain. A laparoscopy is a visual examination inside the abdomen and involves inserting a small viewing instrument into the abdominal cavity through a small incision in the wall of the abdomen. The examination produced minimal findings—nothing that would explain her pain. She was given some painkillers, but the problem did not disappear and continued to bother her more and more. Joy had become more concerned and had further scanning tests. While waiting for the results, she came to me for consultation about some office work. I notice that she was in pain and asked her about it.

I had seen this type of pain before and had relieved it with water. I had used water as a diagnostic test to differentiate between genuine appendicitis pain and dehydration pain that mimics appendicitis. I had written about it in my editorial article, reporting my new method of treating peptic ulcer disease in the June 1983 issue of the *Journal of Clinical Gastroenterology*. I asked Joy to drink a glass of water. Her pain diminished within minutes. The pain disappeared completely when she drank the second glass of water. It had not come back in days. She increased her daily water intake to successfully avoid the pain. Women with pain in their lower abdomen, who have been diagnosed with pain-producing ovarian cysts, inflammation of the fallopian tubes, or even fibroids, should test the authenticity of their diagnosis with one or two glasses of water. It may well be that they are only thirsty and their bodies are only crying for water in that particular region.

AUTOIMMUNE DISEASES

Many degenerative conditions that we do not understand are labeled "autoimmune diseases." It literally means the body is attacking itself without a good cause—at least a cause that should be clear to us in medicine. And since we have never understood dehydration to be as a disease-producing state of body physiology, we have never come across a simple and natural solution to this category of conditions—at least until now. I studied one of these conditions, which has received the label of "lupus," and published my findings in the book *ABC of Asthma, Allergies and Lupus*. I explained why I believe autoimmune diseases should be viewed as conditions produced by persistent unintentional dehydration and its metabolic complications.

In dehydration, and the use of some essential elements as antioxidants to neutralize toxic waste that cannot be excreted because of low urine production, there comes a time when certain vital elements become scarce within the body reserves. However, some of the less vital components of the body have these elements in their assimilated forms. These tissues need to give up some of their precious elements for use in other parts of the body. The whole process is based on priorities and the importance of the elements that are scarce. Under these circumstances and in this category of conditions, the body is forced into a cannibalistic state of physiology. Such cannibalism can cause autoimmune diseases, such as lupus.

The chemical controllers in the body begin to

break down certain tissues to compensate for the missing elements the body needs—especially in the brain. The body always puts the brain first. For example, when the insulin-producing cells of the pancreas are fragmented and destroyed, not only will the ensuing diabetes increase the level of sugar in circulation for the brain to use, but the process will also dehydrate the other tissues of the body and make their water content available for the needs of the brain and the nervous system.

There are some neurological conditions that follow the same logic, such as multiple sclerosis, Alzheimer's disease, muscular dystrophy, Parkinson's disease, and Lou Gehrig's disease (amyotrophic lateral sclerosis). They will be explained in chapter 10, which deals with the brain. AIDS is another condition that I believe finds a better logic as an autoimmune disease, rather than a viral disease, within the discipline of physiology.

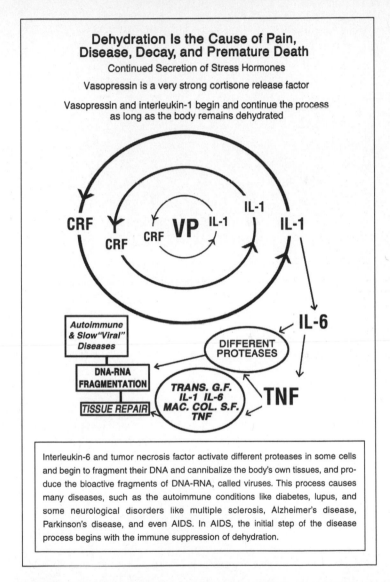

Figure 7.4: A schematic presentation of the sequence of events in water regulation of the body at times of severe dehydration.

CHAPTER 8

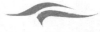

THE CRISIS CALLS OF THE BODY
FOR WATER

The third category of conditions that denote local dehydration are the major pains of the body. Before dehydration hurts you irreversibly, when your plumlike cells become prunelike, your body will show its urgent need for water through different types of pain. These pains are the newly understood, drastic ways of showing dehydration.

After much clinical and scientific research, my understanding is that the early indicators of acid burns in the interior of the cells and potential genetic damage that can take place are different forms and intensities of pain. Depending on the degree of dehydration, as well as the extent and the location of acid buildup inside the cells—when greater flow of water should have cleared the acid from that area—the classic pains of the body are produced. They are:

1. Heartburn
2. Dyspeptic pain
3. Anginal pain

4. Lower back pain
5. Rheumatoid joint pain, including ankylosing spondylitis
6. Migraine headaches
7. Colitis pain
8. Fibromyalgic pains
9. Morning sickness during pregnancy
10. Bulimia

Today, there are 110 million Americans who, at certain times, need pain medications to make life bearable. How pain that is not caused by injury or infection can be produced by dehydration is simple to understand. This very simple mechanism of pain production has eluded us in medicine ever since humankind looked for a way to deal with some of the devastating pains of the human body. The drug industry spends billions of dollars researching painkillers, and even more money advertising their particular brand of pain medication. I don't believe the answer is in these medications, however. Dehydration can be cured by water, for free.

PAIN

To understand the mechanism of pain production in the body, we first need to learn about the way the acid–alkaline balance in the body works. An acidic environment causes irritation of certain nerve endings in the body. When this irritation occurs, the brain is alerted about the chemical environmental change, which is translated and manifested as pain to the conscious mind. In other words, it is the acidity in the interior of the body that causes pain.

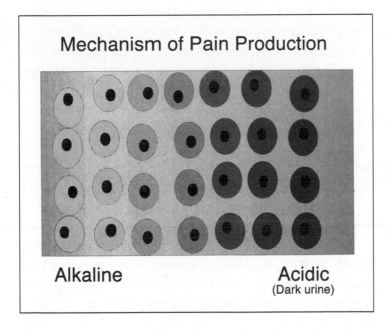

Figure 8.1: Nerve endings register the chemical environmental change with the brain. The brain translates the information for the conscious mind in the form of pain.

Normally, when blood that contains an ample amount of water circulates around the cells of the body, some of the water goes into the cells and brings out hydrogen molecules. Water washes the acidity out of the cell and makes the cell interior alkaline—an absolutely essential and normal state. For optimum health, the body should maintain an alkaline state— pH 7.4 is the desired level.

Why 7.4, and what is pH? The relationship between acid and alkaline is scientifically measured on a scale of 1 to 14. This scale is known as pH. From 1 to 7 on this scale is the acid range, 1 being more acid than 7. From 7 to 14 on the scale is the alkaline range; 7 is less alkaline than 14. On the pH scale, 7 is neutral, meaning optimum. Thus, pH 7.4 of the interior of the cell denotes its natural, slightly alkaline state. This state promotes health because it is the state that best suits the enzymes that function inside the cell: They achieve optimum efficiency at this pH. Adequate flow of water in and out of the cell keeps the cell interior in its health-maintaining, alkaline state.

You have probably seen historic monuments and buildings with artistic statues and carved masonry that have been damaged by pigeons perching on them and smearing them with their droppings. Bird excrement is highly acidic and eats into the stone. In time, the statues and carvings lose their features and definition. The DNA in the nucleus inside the cells of the body is alkaline and, like stone buildings, is also sensitive to the corrosive effects of acidity.

In our bodies, the kidneys mop up excess hydrogen ions—which cause acidity—from the blood and excrete them through the urine that is formed. The more urine that is produced, the more easily the body keeps its interior alkaline. This is why clear urine is an indicator of an efficient acid-clearing mechanism, and dark yellow or orange urine is an ominous sign of impending acid burns in the interior of the body. People who consider having to pass urine more than two or three times a day inconvenient, and do not drink water so that they do not have to urinate more than they can help, are ignorant of how they are hurting their bodies.

The brain is better protected against acid buildup by the fact that it gets priority for delivery of water for all its needs. The rest of the body may not be so fortunate when dehydration establishes in the body and settles in one or another part for a long period of time. With persistent dehydration, however, the brain, too, becomes damaged from acidity in the cells—hence conditions such as Alzheimer's disease, multiple sclerosis, and Parkinson's disease.

Some Specific Pains of Dehydration

As has been explained in the preceding chapters, a large number of medical conditions are caused by the fact that we become unknowingly dehydrated until the body begins to manifest its water shortage in some bizarre but unmistakable ways. Naturally, it is not possible to address all of the ramifications of the many "dis-eases" of the human body that are produced by dehydration in one book. However, I will try to explain some of the more prevalent ones—beginning with the gastrointestinal pains—in sufficient detail as to leave no doubt in your mind that dehydration is their cause.

HEARTBURN OR DYSPEPTIC PAINS

Heartburn or dyspeptic pains are among the most important thirst pains of the human body. Heartburn is the early stage of a gradually intensifying pain that is called dyspeptic pain and eventually peptic ulcer pain. It is felt in the upper part of the abdomen. It can reach an intensity that can incapacitate the person and mimic an acute crisis that requires surgery. Dyspeptic pains, labeled "gastritis," "duodenitis," "esophagitis," "heartburn," and "indigestion after eating," should be treated by only an increase in water intake. When there is associated tissue damage or ulceration, changes to the daily diet that enhance the rate of repair of the ulcer site become necessary. In the above advanced stages of local damage, dyspeptic pain is still a direct signal of dehydration. The ulceration is the product of a protein metabolism disturbance caused by the same stressful and long-lasting dehydration.

In the same way we recognize our hunger pain, the human body also has a thirst pain. We almost always confuse our thirst pain for a signal of food shortage—hence overeating. When this same signal follows a meal, we call it dyspepsia or heartburn, and sufferers are often urged by their doctors and the media to take some form of medication to relieve the pain. After a number of years from the onset of this upper abdominal pain, depending on many other factors, an ulcer may develop. In the interim, the health state is classified as gastritis or duodenitis, until the ulcer develops.

In recent years, because a bacterium called helicobacter is sometimes found in the site of ulcerations, the ulcerations are assumed to be infectious in origin and are treated with antibiotics. However, helicobacter has been recognized to be part of the natural flora—a healthy bacterium—and it lives in the intestines of almost all animals. It seems not to cause an infection in host animals. Labeling peptic ulcer disease as an "infectious condition," in my opinion, provides another opportunity for commercialism in medicine to thrive.

Because we do not recognize heartburn as a signal of body thirst, its significance is not understood until an ulcer develops. However, the consequences of this chronic dehydration do not confine themselves to the stomach and intestine. There are many associated health problems that will gradually reveal themselves. Everyone should be alert to heartburn as a major thirst pain of the body, which can occur at all ages.

In some, the sensation of thirst may not at first be signaled by severe pain; it may initially be felt as a discomfort in the upper part of the abdomen. In others, the pain may be so severe that an inexperienced clinician might think of it as indicative of a surgical condition and may even perform exploratory surgery and not find any physical sign of a disease. Sometimes the pain is felt around the appendix area and mimics appendicitis. Physicians should consider this type of thirst pain signal when making a diagnosis associated with lower abdominal pains. In some people, the severe pain might be felt on the left side, over the large intestine, and is often identified as colitis. This pain, too, should initially be considered as a thirst signal. If it is not relieved after one or two glasses of water, and not completely gone in a few days of increased water intake, then other local pathology may have to be investigated. It must be remembered that it takes a few days of increased daily water intake before chronic cellular dehydration can be partially reduced.

The conscious mind has a problem with recognizing the body's water needs. Full and adequate hydration of the body depends on the sharpness of its thirst perception. Unfortunately, as it ages, the body gradually loses its ability to recognize its dehydration. Elderly people can become chronically dehydrated, even if there is plenty of drinking water available, because they fail to recognize their extreme thirst. The more the body becomes dehydrated, the more the brain's water-regulating chemicals—histamine and its subordinate local officers—become engaged in their water-shunting and -rationing responsibilities.

A Typical Case History

J. B., a company administrative secretary, developed peptic ulcer disease when she was thirty-three years old. The usual medications—antacids that neutralize the acid in the stomach—could not give relief. Stronger prescription medications (which are actually very strong histamine-blocking agents that temporarily stop acid production in the stomach) would at best partially relieve her symptoms of severe dyspeptic pain. On and off, the disease recurred several times a year for a number of years. On a number of occasions, she had to seek her doctor's advice for her stress and ulcer pains on a weekly basis.

A few years ago, during one of these periods of persistent stomach pains that seemed reluctant to yield to the effect of very strong medications, her doctor—with much caution—told her that severe peptic ulcer pain seemed to have been satisfactorily relieved with ordinary tap water. J. B. was encouraged to increase her water intake anytime she developed stomach pain to see is this could be effective. The treatment worked. For a number of years now, J. B. has followed this advice. With the slightest indication of her pain coming back, an increase in her daily intake of water makes it disappear. As a result of a program of drinking eight glasses of water a day, J. B. no longer suffers from ulcer pains. She has no more need for any medication other than the water she now drinks regularly to prevent the pains from recurring.

The explanation for the occurrence of heartburn as a signal of water deficiency is very simple. When we drink water, it is immediately passed into the intestine and absorbed. It seems that, within a half hour, it is once again secreted into the stomach from the base of the dents in the mucosa. One of the major events that take place is a backwash of the mucus layer that expands and stores naturally secreted bicarbonate that neutralizes the acid on its surface.

For the cells under it, the mucus layer lining the stomach is a protective insulation against the acid, which is poured on food for the process of digestion. This backwash of the mucus by the water we drink is an essential part of the maintenance of the protective system of the stomach wall. Water flowing through the mucus layer brings about the expansion and thick-

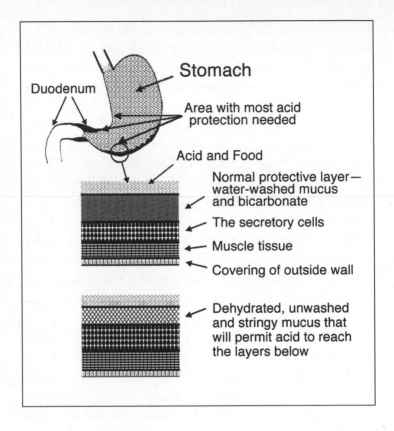

Figure 8.2: Schematic drawing of the shape of the stomach and its mucus layer. A hydrated mucus barrier is uniform in consistency and prevents acid penetration. Dehydrated mucus becomes stringy and allows acid penetration.

ening of this protective layer in the stomach. Mucus is 98 percent water and 2 percent scaffolding that holds the water in place. The water in turn dissolves the bicarbonate that acts as the buffer for the acid that will try to pass through the mucus. This is a constantly active process. Dehydration alters the consistency of the mucus barrier, rendering it ineffective as a buffer against the acid in the stomach. It allows the acid to go through and reach the cells below, thus causing pain—"heartburn."

HIATAL HERNIA AND HEARTBURN

A dome-shaped muscle called the diaphragm separates the chest cavity from the abdomen. It is attached to the rib cage and to some of the lower vertebrae of the spine. At the back of the diaphragm, where it is attached to the spine, is an opening through which the esophagus and the main blood vessels pass. This opening is called the hiatus and it acts as a "purse-string" gate. It is composed of a band of overlapping muscle that keeps the gate closed. It relaxes only when food is passing through the esophagus in the chest cavity to enter the stomach, which is normally positioned below the diaphragm in the abdomen. The automatic opening and closing of the gate is synchronized with the flow of food through the esophagus. When food is not passing through, the gate is closed and the chest cavity is well separated from the abdomen and its contents. In some people, the gate becomes lax and its opening less firm. In these people, the upper part of the stomach may bulge or become herniated through the hiatus and shift into the chest cavity—hence hiatal hernia. The reason why the hiatal gate becomes lax is chronic dehydration.

From its opening in the mouth to the orifice of the

rectum, the intestinal tract is a long tube that has developed special characteristics in different segments along its length. The intestinal tract works like a conveyor belt that pushes its contents downstream. The intestinal tract can also reverse the direction of its waves and push its contents upward. This process is involved when the contents of the stomach must not go downstream and must be forced out of the body— heralded by nausea and then vomiting.

The esophagus is a long tube that carries food and fluids into the stomach, which is situated in the abdomen. The stomach is a pouch that produces acid and protein-breaking enzymes that liquefy the solid foods we eat. The duodenum is the segment of the small intestine that connects to the stomach and is separated from it by a special gate called the pyloric valve. In the duodenum, the pancreatic enzymes are secreted along with a watery bicarbonate solution to further digest the liquefied food from the stomach and neutralize the acid that gets into the intestine. The stomach has a protective mucus coating on its mucosa that prevents the acid from damaging it (figure 8.2). The duodenum does not have the same protective mucus coating to defend it against the acid from the stomach. It depends on the watery bicarbonate secretion from the pancreas to do the job. In dehydration, the quantity of the watery bicarbonate solution made by the pancreas is insufficient to deal with all the acid that is going to reach the duodenum. There comes a point where, if the entire acidic contents of the stomach were to enter the small intestine (the duodenum), its mucosa would be irreparably damaged.

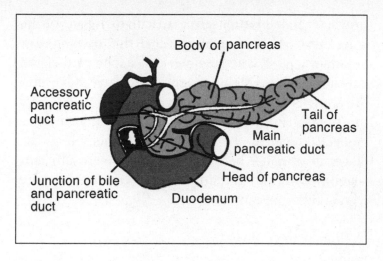

Figure 8.3: Pancreas where watery bicarbonate solution is manufactured and secreted into duodenum.

Inside the pyloric valve are sensors—like spokes of a wheel that stick out when the stomach contents are passed into the duodenum—that register the consistency and the acidity of the stomach contents. Only if the acidity of the stomach contents can be neutralized completely by the amount of the alkaline secretion from the pancreas will the pyloric valve open and allow the stomach contents to enter the intestine. What goes through is proportionate to the amount that can be neutralized. At a crisis stage of dehydration, when heartburn or dyspeptic pain is also produced, the high acidity in the stomach cannot go into the intestine. It cannot stay in the stomach for long, either.

In this situation, some of the acidic contents of the

stomach can bubble upward, particularly when you are lying down. This is when you feel the discomfort of heartburn. At the same time, the upper part of the stomach can also slide through the hiatal valve into the chest cavity. You might have to vomit to get rid of the stomach contents, or get sufficient antacid treatment to suppress the symptoms. Nonetheless, the diagnosis of hiatal hernia will stick. Given sufficient water every day, the situation can reverse itself and the pain and hernia can disappear.

Bulimia

I am sure you are very sympathetic to people who have been given the label of "bulimic." These people eat and then throw up whatever they have eaten. The most famous bulimic was probably the late Princess Diana. Bulimia sufferers are constantly hungry, and are also depressed and antisocial, as seems to have been the case with Princess Diana throughout her private and married life.

There is a belief among pundits who profess to understand bulimia, that the whole problem is caused by an undercurrent of psychological issues within the thought processes of bulimics. Since more women suffer from the problem than men, it is assumed that the act of eating and then throwing up whatever has been eaten is a measure to remain thin. I disagree.

Uncontrollable and repeated vomiting of the stomach contents, which has been given the medical labels of "heartburn" or "bulimia," could be one of the ways the body prevents irreparable damage when it is severely dehydrated. When it is said that bulimics feel hungry all the time, there is confusion. As far as I am concerned, they are confusing their sensation of thirst with the sensation of hunger. When they should be drinking water, they eat. Naturally, the body rejects the food because it does not possess enough water to digest and assimilate the food. This is the reason why bulimics grow so thin. The same dehydration can also be responsible for some of the emotional and psychological changes in these people.

I met Amir in the prison where I started to research the impact of water on the treatment of peptic ulcer disease. For more than ten years, on and off, he had been suffering from heartburn. During the flare-up phase of the problem, he would routinely vomit in his sleep—so forcefully that part of his stomach contents would jet out of his nose. Often he could not clear out of his bed in time to avoid making a mess. You can imagine he had difficulty sleeping during these times. Because none of the regular medications could stop such vomiting, he had taken it for granted that his problem was incurable.

I asked him to drink a full glass of water a half hour before his food and increase his daily water intake. As simply as you read these lines, his heartburn disappeared and never came back while he was in the prison with me.

Let me share with you the human side of Amir's story. It is interesting that in his immediate family, his daughter, his wife, and his brother had similar problems—heartburn that culminated in vomiting when the disease flared up. At this time in the life of the family, when there was a lot of fear that Amir might not get out of prison anytime soon, none of them was in a good state of health. They were stressed beyond words. They would travel for miles every week to see Amir. They would wait outside the prison walls for hours, in the heat of the summer and the cold of the winter, to have a ten- to fifteen-minute visitation.

On one of these occasions, he shared with them the fact that increased water intake had cured him of his "disease." He was jubilant that now his family could do the same. One by one they got rid of their devastating heartburn and the social complications of the problem they had experienced for many years. Luck was with Amir. He was released unexpectedly. Before he left, he came to me and thanked me for what I had done for him. He told me, "It was worth coming to prison to get cured of my disease."

The Danger of Antacids

Antacids that contain aluminum can be dangerous. They should not be freely used for dyspepsia that responds simply to an increase in water intake. Excess aluminum in the circulation has been strongly implicated as a precipitating factor in Alzheimer's-type diseases. It is imperative to understand the relationship between taking antacids for a long period and their possible toxic side effects, the local brain damage and plaques seen in Alzheimer's disease a number of years later. Plaques are tangled masses of tissue that contain high aluminum deposits. Fortunately, the drug industry in America is now producing some antacids that do not contain aluminum.

Zinc is a very important metal for genetic transcription and manufacture of important hormones and brain chemicals. Metals have a special transport system across cell membranes. If aluminum is carried across into brain cells in place of zinc, much damage will occur. Although the body can repair and replace cells in most tissues or organs, brain cells are not regenerated or replaced. They die and leave a cyst, or are replaced by fibrous tissue—the sort of pathology seen in Alzheimer's disease.

The older antacids on the market contained between 60 and 150 milligrams of aluminum per spoonful of the liquid. It had been assumed the body cannot absorb this metal; it acts locally in the stomach. However, the fact that aluminum is found in high concentration in the brain tissue of those suffering from Alzheimer's disease should make us aware that a high intake of aluminum over a long period can lead to some absorption of the metal—enough to cause damage at some point.

When the body becomes gradually dehydrated as a result of the loss of its thirst sensation, to the extent that it develops dyspeptic pain as a thirst signal, many of the functions of the body are already affected. The most affected is the brain itself. Although the brain cells themselves are fully developed, the nerve system—the "wire works"—can become damaged in dehydration. The most affected part will be the connection points in the wire system. There is much regeneration going on at these interconnections, which are constantly used. In Alzheimer's disease, these interconnections are tangled, and a great deal of aluminum seems to be deposited at these points.

Another problem in most neurological disorders—such as multiple sclerosis (MS), Parkinson's disease, and Lou Gehrig's disease (amyotrophic lateral sclerosis)—seen on MRI brain scans is widespread plaques over the brain tissue. This phenomenon will be explained later in the book.

In Guam, where many aluminum deposits are to be found in the soil, the drinking water at one time had high levels of aluminum contamination. During this time, an Alzheimer's-type disease was prevalent on the island, with even the younger population being affected. When the aluminum contamination was removed from the source of drinking water, the rate of Alzheimer's-type disease among the population decreased. Thus, there seems to be a correlation between Alzheimer's-type disease and aluminum poisoning.

The Disadvantages of Antihistamine Medications

It has been learned that histamine production is involved in allergies and pain. The opportunity to immediately commercialize this significant finding has resulted in the production of a number of different antihistamine medications. Histamine, however, is an agent that has many useful functions. It operates the main brain sensory system for water intake, distribution, and rationing. It is also a strong regulator of energy expenditure in the body. When the body is well supplied with water, the activity of histamine is confined to its local actions of shunting the circulation to bring water to the more active parts of the body, especially the central nervous system.

If the brain has to be very active and needs more circulation, histamine kicks into action. This can have the effect of producing acid in the stomach, causing heartburn, a primary thirst signal. Antihistamines, which temporarily suppress the pain-producing action of histamine in the intestinal tract, will over time cause damage because they do not correct for the basic problem of dehydration. At the same time, antihistamines can suppress brain activity. They also reduce libido and can cause some male hormonal imbalance and enlargement of the breasts in men. In the elderly, they may cause confusion and disorientation.

Pain, at first, is a peripheral marker of thirst. Ultimately, and if allowed to continue, pain becomes the main brain marker for the same thirst. At the early phase of pain, some substances may blunt the peripheral marker and silence the thirst signal, such as antacids, food, or even histamine-blocking agents. But at a certain threshold of dehydration, the brain-initiated pain is not fooled by the action of locally acting medication, food, or indeed anything other than water that must be delivered into the stomach.

Let me tell you the story of a young man. This case stands out as an example of the brain marker for dehydration of the body. I reported this case in my editorial article in the *Journal of Clinical Gastroenterology* in June 1983. I have seen a number of similar cases.

I had the occasion to visit late one evening a young man in his twenties. He had a long history of peptic ulcer disease. Ten hours earlier, he had developed classic upper abdominal pain. His symptoms became more severe as time passed. He had taken almost a full bottle of antacid and three Tagamet tablets with no effect. The pain persisted. When I saw him, he was in such severe pain that he lay on the floor of the room curled up, groaning, eyes shut, and not alert to his environment. He seemed to be semiconscious. When I spoke to him, he did not seem to hear. I had to shake him to get a response. When I asked him what was the matter, he told me: "My ulcer is killing me." I examined him for a perforated ulcer, which fortunately he did not have. I made him drink two large glasses of water. It took him about ten minutes to feel some relief. A third glass of water was given to him fifteen minutes after the first two drinks. By now he was obviously in much less pain. Twenty minutes after the initial intake of water he had recovered completely, to the point that he sat up and began talking to the people around him.

This patient and his friends had observed the pain-relieving miracles hidden in a glassful of water. The clinical evaluation of this case indicates that the human body has a central nervous system pain signal for water deficiency. In the past, many such cases must have ended up on the operating tables of overzealous surgeons (I am sure some still do). It was also my experience and observation that some of these centrally produced pains for thirst occur in the area of the appendix, on the lower right side of the abdomen. I have had occasion to demonstrate the diagnostic value of a glass of water in doubtful and atypical cases of pain in the lower parts of the abdomen, such as in the case of Joy on page 119.

Eventually a dehydration-induced dyspeptic pain signal may graduate to a more advanced stage of complication, involving tryptophan. Tryptophan is an essential amino acid of the body (discussed under essential amino acids in chapter 14). In prolonged dehydration, it seems to become depleted from the body reserves. This amino acid is a prominent player in the repair systems of the body, as well as being the primary material for formation of a number of neurotransmitters that also suppress pain. If water by itself does not alleviate dyspeptic pain, an alteration in diet to increase the intake of natural foods that contain sufficient tryptophan for the needs of the body becomes essential. For more detail, read the section on tryptophan.

COLITIS PAIN

The origin of this pain was discussed in the section on constipation in chapter 7. There is no harm in saying a few words here, now that we are discussing the major pains of the body. Pain in the left lower region of the abdomen, often identified as colitis pain, seems to respond to an increase in daily water intake. Water plays an integral role in the digestion process. For the final products of food digestion to pass through the intestine, the lubricating property of water is essential. At the same time, the lower region of the large intestine in particular is responsible for final absorption of water from the excrement. This process becomes more operative at the time of dehydration. There is a central control for the peristaltic contractions of the intestine at the time of food digestion and its passage through the intestine. When there is dehydration, the normal peristalsis is reduced and a tighter contraction to squeeze the water from the solid matter seems to become necessary. This process causes pain. If two or three glasses of water are taken, particularly first thing in the morning, the pain should disappear, if the original cause of pain is dehydration and not other, more serious, conditions. At the same time, the associated constipation should subside and movement of the bowels will become regular and normal.

HEADACHES AND MIGRAINE

As mentioned, the brain is very sensitive to the dehydration and heat regulation of the body. The brain cannot endure overheating. Its enzyme systems are very sensitive to temperature fluctuations. When there is water shortage in the body and there is potential for getting dehydrated or getting overheated because of too many bedcovers at night, the brain establishes a priority for itself, at the expense of the other tissues of the body. It allows more blood to flow through its vascular system. The blood vessels to the brain—the carotid arteries—take root from the main artery of the heart, the aorta. The carotid arteries supply blood to the scalp, face, and tongue before they pass into the skull to supply the brain. When the command for increased supply of blood to the brain forces these arteries to dilate, the circulation to the face and the scalp also increases. This is the reason why some headaches begin with strongly pulsating arteries around the temples.

The brain capillary system is under the direct influence of histamine on its receptors. Histamine, apart from its direct water-regulatory responsibilities to the brain, is also involved in temperature regulation of the body. It has two cooling functions. It lowers the core temperature of the body and is also involved in facilitating perspiration and sweating to help cool the body.

Histamine that is released because of the brain's concern for its dehydration or overheating activates certain systems to promote more circulation to correct the problem. When there is dehydration in the brain area—whether it is caused by insufficient intake of water, stress, alcohol, or overheating of the body—the action of histamine causes the pain we know as a headache or migraine. To alleviate this type of pain, two, three, even four glasses of water may have to be taken. The water should be cool in order to allow a better circulation of the diluted blood to the brain area. It is interesting to note that all normal painkillers cut the connection between histamine and one of its major subordinate systems. It is my understanding that migraine is a centrally produced signal for dehydration and overheating of the brain. This is the reason most painkillers do not work for migraine headaches.

RHEUMATOID ARTHRITIS PAIN

The separation of lower back pain from rheumatoid joint pains elsewhere in the body is inaccurate. The mechanism of pain production in these joint conditions seems to be the same. They denote the same physiological phenomenon in the body. The separation of these two problems in the medical industry seems to be a matter of convenience for the involvement of different subspecialties. For the one, you go to a rheumatologist; for the other, to an orthopedic surgeon or chiropractor. The outcome is the same—pain management rather than a cure. Basically, both conditions have the same pathology, except they are in different locations.

About fifty million Americans—two hundred thousand of them children—are said to suffer some sort of arthritis pain, and some thirty million suffer back pain. Each year a few million are said to be functionally disabled from back pain. In the United States, it is estimated that sixteen billion dollars is spent annually on back pain treatment, and a further eighty billion dollars is lost in productivity and wages as a result of back pain. These commonly quoted statistics, even if partially accurate, indicate a devastating problem for the American people.

New Insight into the Phenomenon of Joint Pains

In chronically painful joint conditions of the lower spine or joints of the hands and legs, the actual recurring pain is a signal of water deficiency in the area where pain is felt. The pain occurs because there is not enough water circulation to wash out local acidity and toxic substances. These regional joint pains are part of a series of newly understood crisis thirst signals of the body. Where the pain is felt depends on where the localized drought has settled in.

Lower back pain has two components: one, muscle spasm (this is the cause of 80 percent of back pains); two, disc degeneration that puts added strain on the tendons and ligaments in the spinal column. Both of these back-pain-causing conditions are initiated by the same chronic dehydration. With the new information about the emergency calls of the body for water, there is no reason why back and joint pains should continue to devastate our bodies. We now have the insight and knowledge about why these pains occur, and how to *prevent* them. More detailed information on these two topics is available in my book *How to Deal with Back Pain and Rheumatoid Joint Pain* and my videotape *How to Deal with Back Pain*.

All joint surfaces possess cartilage padding, which covers and separates the bone structures in the joint. This firm layer of cartilage contains a vast quantity of water, which provides it with the ability to glide over the opposing cartilage surface and aids the necessary lubrication for the joint movements. Thus, prolonged dehydration that leaves the cartilage short of water will produce a greater friction and shearing stress at the cartilage contact points in the joint.

Intelligence Behind the Design of the Body

When cartilage is dehydrated, its gliding ability is decreased. The cartilage cells sense their dehydration and give out alarm signals of pain, because they would soon die and peel off from their contact surfaces of the bones if used in their dehydrated state. The normal environment of cartilage is alkaline. In dehydration, it becomes acidic. This acidity sensitizes the nerve endings that register pain. This type of pain has to be treated with a regular increase in water intake until the cartilage is fully hydrated and washed of its acidity and toxins. Often the pain travels from joint to joint; sometimes it appears in the corresponding joints in the other limb at the same time. Chronic pains have two components: peripheral and brain-generated pains. Locally initiated pain is relieved by analgesics, such as aspirin or Tylenol, but brain-level pain is not. Both pains are relieved by the intake of adequate water.

Cartilage is a gelatinous living tissue; its cells like to live in an alkaline environment. The alkalinity of the medium depends on the amount of water that flows through the cartilage to wash the acid away. Salt helps extract the acidity from inside the cartilage cells and pass it into the water, which carries the acid away. This is a constant process. For this process to be effective, two elements are vital: water and salt. Adequate salt supply is essential for the prevention of arthritis pain, be it in the joints of the limbs or the spine. It is the salt level in the serum that increases the fluid volume for its more abundant flow through the cartilage.

What Happens to a Dehydrated Joint?

Cartilage cells die at a fast pace because of the constant abrasive friction in the dehydrated joint. These cells need to be replaced. When there is damage to the cartilage because of its overuse and under-repair, the sensors in the area begin to indicate a desperate need for urgent repair. An attempt is made to supply water to the cartilage cells from the blood supply. This action supplies some lubrication inside the joint, but is not effective in maintaining the rate of cartilage growth to replace the dead tissue. In the lining of the joint capsule are cells that can secrete local hormones to stimulate repair activity at the same time that they begin to produce pain. Several things happen when these hormones are secreted:

1. The dying tissue is broken up from inside the cells and the broken fragments are extruded. They are ingested by white cells—the "garbage collectors"— and are recycled.

2. More blood circulation is brought to the affected area, and this results in swelling and stretching in the joint capsule, which causes stiffness and, eventually, added pain.
3. There is an associated protein breakdown, and more amino acids are mobilized for the pool that may be needed for the repair of the damage.
4. In the inflammatory environment inside the joint, some white cells begin to manufacture hydrogen peroxide and ozone for two purposes: one, to keep the joint space sterilized and to prevent bacteria from infecting the joint cavity; two, to supply with adequate oxygen the cells that are engaged in the repair process and have less access to the blood oxygen.
5. There is a local remodeling growth factor that promotes the growth of tissue, causing the typical gnarled joints of arthritis.
6. Knowledge gained by the brain from its ongoing experience is put to use for the rest of the body. The remodeling and fortification—gnarling, deformity—of other similarly structured joints will also be carried out. This seems to be the reason rheumatoid joints of the hands show a mirror-image inflammation and eventual gnarling of the joints on both sides.

LOWER BACK PAIN

As mentioned earlier, lower back pain has two components—muscle spasm that causes pain, and disc degeneration that puts strain on the tendons and ligaments in the spinal column. Lower back pain indicates exactly the same problem that was explained regarding rheumatoid joint pains of the hands, except the circulation system to the spinal disc space is difficult, and the disc core depends on the creation of an intermittent vacuum in the disc space. This natural process is a component of the walking movement. Of course, the body must be well-hydrated for water to leave the circulation and enter the disc spaces.

In the spinal column, the weight of the body is supported by twenty-three discs and twenty-four vertebrae. The discs are housed between plates of cartilage that cover opposing flat surfaces of the vertebrae. The end-plate cartilage attached to its flat weight-bearing surfaces is part of the structure of each vertebra. During the movement of each vertebra, the disc is meant to glide minimally between the end-plate cartilage located on its upper and lower surfaces. Seventy-five percent of the weight of the upper body mass is supported by the hydraulic properties of the discs that absorb and hold water in their central cores. In a dehydrated state, when the body mass constantly squeezes out the water content of the discs during movement and bending, not enough of the lost water can be replaced. The dehydrated discs with their shrunken cores gradually become less supportive of the weight of the body. The discs lose their wedge quality, and the spinal joints become less firm. In a well-hydrated and taut state, on the other hand, the discs themselves do not physically move, but get continuously squeezed of water and then, through force of vacuum, absorb water again and expand to function as the natural shock absorbers they are designed to be.

In a dehydrated state, the discs can shift backward to press on the local nerves. When this happens in the lower spinal region, the pain becomes projected into one or the other leg. This is called sciatic pain and is far more serious than local pain in the back. It means the spinal joint structure has become so disorganized that one of the discs that has to shock-absorb for the spine is out of its normal position and is pressing on the nerve. Dehydration and bad posture are involved in this condition. For more information, and to learn a new technique for the reduction of the disc displacement and relief from sciatic pain, I encourage you to refer to my book *How to Deal with Back Pain and Rheumatoid Joint Pain*.

OSTEOARTHRITIS

When the cartilage in the joint dies, bone-to-bone contact begins. Whereas cartilage cells have a water-given resilience and can survive the trauma of movement against one another, the hardened bone surfaces produce a friction force against one another. This friction force produces an inflammatory process that destroys the bone surfaces. Thus osteoarthritis of the joint occurs—a second-stage process to dehydration that first destroys the cartilage surfaces.

Given that osteoarthritis sufferers are so often prescribed painkillers—acetaminophen, ibuprofen, and aspirin—I found this recent article particularly interesting. "Link Suggested in Hypertension and Painkillers" is the title given by the *New York Times* of October 28, 2002, to a report on an article published in the *Archive of Internal Medicine* by a group from Harvard Medical School. The study involved more than eighty thousand women between the ages of thirty-one and fifty, who participated in a nurses' health study and were not known to have high blood pressure at the outset. These people were using painkillers since 1995 and their blood pressures were obtained from a survey two years later. In the two years, 1,650 women had developed hypertension. Women who used acetaminophen (present in Tylenol) and ibuprofen (sold under many different names, including Motrin and Brufen) as their painkiller were 86 percent more susceptible to develop hypertension than the nonusers of these brands of pain medication. The article seems to whitewash aspirin and did not involve it in causing hypertension.

I have no idea who funded the research and which company stands to gain from the results of this study. I am perturbed by the shameful limitation of knowledge that exists at one of the most prestigious medical schools in the world—Harvard University—about the variety of ways the human body manifests dehydration. The researchers who conducted the study are oblivious to the fact that pain is one of the crisis calls of the body for water, and that hypertension is the body's adaptive process to the same dehydration—one of its drought-management programs. They do not realize that hypertension and pain are different proclamations of the same problem: water shortage in the body. All that painkillers do is mask one of the localized signals of dehydration until hypertension, the next indicator of generalized drought, reveals itself.

I believe that this is scientifically a more accurate conclusion to the above study: Go and take water, and do *not* go and take aspirin in preference to acetaminophen. Reading this book, you will be able to see this logic. Who knows, in the future you might even be in a position to save many people from their very drastic health problems with this simple information.

CHAPTER 9

DEHYDRATION AND DISEASE

The following conditions are produced by persistent dehydration in the fourth dimension, time: the time it takes for the damage to slowly erode the body, emerge, and show itself in a characteristic way that can be identified and labeled according to various symptoms we routinely come across. These conditions (states of dehydration) have been labeled "diseases of unknown origin" by the mainstream medical establishment. Creation of jargons around different ways the body shows it is dehydrated seems to have given the mainstream medical establishment license to treat these manifestations of dehydration with bizarre and unnecessary protocols. Some of these conditions include:

1. Obesity
2. Raised low-density cholesterol in the blood circulation
3. Raised triglycerides
4. Cholesterol plaque formation in the arteries
5. Coronary thrombosis
6. Osteoporosis

7. Osteoarthritis
8. Heart failure
9. Repeated strokes
10. Juvenile diabetes
11. Alzheimer's disease
12. Multiple sclerosis
13. Amyotrophic lateral sclerosis, otherwise known as Lou Gehrig's disease
14. Muscular dystrophy
15. Parkinson's disease
16. Scleroderma
17. Cancers
18. AIDS

What has been discovered for the first time in the history of modern science-based medicine is the way to prevent and cure degenerative diseases of the human body—simply and naturally with water. The cause of these health problems has been discovered and exposed for everyone's benefit. In short, prevent dehydration to prevent disease!

Some of the conditions listed above have already been discussed.

In this chapter we will discuss obesity. The other topics will be discussed under separate chapters and headings.

OBESITY

A simple solution to obesity is of interest to many, many people. I think if we understand the relationship of overeating to the dehydration of the body, we will also understand how to prevent obesity. The next step is how to reduce the volume of fat that has been deposited. The answer to both these enigmas is simple. To institute the advice, however, you need discipline and determination. It should also be remembered that the metabolism of fat, in a way to reduce many pounds of excess weight, is a slow process if it is to be done without adverse effects to your general health. The most important step in this direction is to build a mental image of a slimmer you. Visualize your body with many pounds off it. Store this image in your sub-conscious mind and keep impressing upon your brain your desire for this outcome.

There are two general sensations associated with eating habits. The one for food is often termed hunger pain. The second is a sensation for thirst. Both are felt in the same area and are brought about by histamine. It is easy to confuse the two signals and to think we are hungry when we are really thirsty. We mistakenly think we are thirsty only when the mouth becomes dry. Relying on the dry mouth stage of dehydration is the basic problem. This signal for water intake is a last-stage situation and is often seen after heavy eating. The best way to separate the sensation of thirst from that of hunger is to drink water before food. In some animal species, this order is maintained. Animals make an early-morning visit to a water source before going into the field for grazing, even when vegetation with high water content is their diet. In humans, the reverse has become a habit. We often first take food and then water—and sometimes only after the body gets thoroughly dehydrated by the intake of solid foods that use up the available free water in the body. This, I believe, is the root cause of obesity.

Obese people consume food to satisfy the initial calls of histamine for water. This is because food is also converted to ATP and is more satisfying to the taste buds than water. To satisfy the brain's needs for ATP, however, water is infinitely more efficient and immediately more effective. With food we can generate energy for brain function only from sugar. However, we consume five times more than the full needs of the brain itself. After all, only about 20 percent of the circulation goes to the brain. The other 80 percent, now laden with sugar, goes to the other organs, including fat cells that store the sugar in the form of fat. The more food we eat, the more sugar will end up as fat, when all the time the brain wanted water to generate hydroelectricity, a clean source of energy.

Over time, this process of histamine response to dehydration, or mental and social stresses of the body, can become the basis for overeating when the initial need of the body is simply water by itself. Thus, dehydration of the body can be the root cause of obesity that is more often than not associated with hypertension and will ultimately lead to diabetes at a later stage. The information on diabetes (see chapter 7) will complement this understanding of obesity.

There is a very simple solution to this problem. A half hour before each meal of the day, and two and a half hours after each meal, drink two glasses of water. It seems to take about a half hour before the physiology in search of water is separated from that of hunger for food. You will feel full and will eat only when food is needed. The volume of food intake will decrease drastically. The type of craving for food will also change. With sufficient water intake, we tend to crave proteins more than fattening carbohydrates.

The next desirable step is the shedding of already gained fat. Increased water intake by itself will begin to reduce some of the gained weight. About eight to fourteen pounds may be lost in less than three weeks. This immediate weight loss will be from the collection of edema fluid that is stored in the tissues to operate the reverse-system of water delivery into vital cells. If, in addition to increased water intake, you activate hormone-sensitive, fat-burning enzymes, the weight loss will be more pronounced and well proportioned.

Gross obesity afflicts 37 percent of the American population. Now even children are getting grossly obese. It is estimated that obesity prematurely kills more than four hundred thousand people every year. Yet this killer disease can be prevented, and even cured, by proper hydration. The reason is simple. Collecting and storing fat is one of the major complications of dehydration. It is caused when the sensation of thirst is confused with the sensation of hunger, and instead of drinking water, the person eats. Brain function prefers to receive clean energy (so to speak) from hydroelectricity. When it is forced to use dirty energy from food, only 20 percent of this energy reaches the brain. Unless used in movement, exercise, or energy-consuming occupations, the rest of the energy from food is stored in the form of fat.

When fat is formed and stored, its breakdown is initiated only by specific chemical commands. Lipase is the enzyme that breaks down fat and converts the lumps into small fatty acid particles that are then used by the muscles and in the liver. Certain hormones that regulate body activity stimulate lipase activity. At the top of the list is adrenaline of the sympathetic nervous system. It has been shown that a glass of water stimulates the sympathetic nervous system for one and a half to two hours. The end result of adrenaline secretion is clearly a gradual loss of stored fat and a dramatic reduction of excess weight. This kind of weight loss is more stable and permanent than other ways of dieting and reducing calorie intake.

The fat-burning enzymes are sensitive to the hormones of physical activity—adrenaline and its family. These hormones are produced when the muscles are active and begin to burn fat as their staple diet—hence the value of regular walks. I have seen some people lose twenty-five to forty-five pounds in a comparatively short period of time through increased water intake and increased regular exercise. I have seen a man lose 290 pounds in one year; another lost 305 pounds in sixteen months. One of them needed two operations to remove the loose skin from his body. You will read testimonials of dramatic weight loss with my protocol. With my approach to weight regulation, not much dieting will be needed. You are free to eat any form of food the body calls for. The body itself becomes selective. All the body sensations become sharp, including the selection sensors that identify the body's needs.

The direct connection between muscle activity and

stimulation of the hormone-sensitive lipase was discovered in Sweden. A few years ago, the Swedish army did a field test on a company of soldiers that was taken on a three-week march. At repeated intervals, blood samples were taken and various tests were done to monitor the impact of marching on the body physiology of the soldiers. They discovered that after an hour's march, the same hormone-sensitive lipase became active and stayed in the circulation for no less than twelve hours. They also discovered that continuous walking had a cumulative effect; the activity of the enzyme could be measured around the clock and in a much more pronounced way. In effect, the outcome of this experiment indicates that two sessions of daily walks would program the body into a round-the-clock fat-burning mode. Thus, walking should always be a part of any weight-loss program. One success story of how water was effective in a dramatic weight-reduction program is presented in the letter below.

Dear Dr. Batman,

For most of my life, I have been overweight. Every family has a "fat child" and this was me. I was told that I was just "big boned" and I should be content with who I was. Then I heard about The Water Cure. I was skeptical at first, because how could drinking iced tea and cola be such a problem? But I thought that all I really had to lose was my weight. Over a period of a year and a half, I have lost approximately 100 pounds and am no longer the "fat kid" that everyone knew.

But besides losing the weight, I have noticed that acid reflux, which had been a major part of my life, was also now gone. I could now enjoy foods that previously had brought me nothing but sickness. I have also noticed that I no longer get ear infections that also seemed commonplace and inevitable problems of life to me at one time.

I also have more energy and feel as if I have become a whole new person. I have energy to do things that would have easily worn me out previously.

Thank you Dr. Batman for helping me!

Losing weight through proper hydration of the body, some salt intake, and exercise is more prudent than drastic dieting. Complications of drastic dieting and of focusing only on the readings of the weight scale can cause an unbalanced intake of essential ingredients and precipitate deficiency diseases. The good thing about water as the primary source of clean energy is the fact that any excess is passed out in the form of urine. Fat, on the other hand, has to be burned through many steps until it is converted to carbon dioxide and passed out in the lungs.

Woman's World Magazine of September 4, 2001, dedicated its cover and two inside pages to a dramatic splash on the weight-loss program of The Water Cure. The headline read, REVOLUTIONARY MEDICAL BREAK-THROUGH, THE SLIMMING NEW WATER CURE! LEARN HOW TO DRINK AWAY 40 LBS. OR MORE! The cover shows a picture of Finola Hughes, star of the television series *All My Children*, who lost thirty pounds without dieting. Among other stories, the article also highlights how a radio talk-show host lost forty pounds without effort and has gone down from a size 20 to a size 14. She not only lost her flab, she also got rid of her hot flashes, fatigue, aching joints, and sinus headaches, all in one sweep.

Unfortunately, the children in America are now showing an astounding tendency to gain weight. This subject has become an issue in the media and within the government. Fat children and adolescents are showing a tendency toward developing the same diseases as grown-ups, such as early-onset type II diabetes, known as adult-onset diabetes. The reason, I believe, is twofold. One, they are being pushed into overeating by the food industry's constant advertising that promotes different fast foods. Two, these children are pushed to drink sweetened drinks instead of water. Any form of sweetness sensed by the tongue will stimulate the pancreas to secrete insulin. Insulin is a weight-gain-promoting (anabolic) hormone; it promotes fat cells to convert sugar and carbohydrates in the diet into fat.

Let me briefly touch on the importance of salt to weight loss. When the body becomes dehydrated and needs to increase its water reserves, it can do so only if salt is available to expand the extracellular water content of the body. In dehydration, the body seeks salt in the foods that are eaten. This search for salt is another reason for overeating.

If ever you wonder about the validity of water as the natural "preventive" medication in staying slim and in avoiding the many diseases listed above, remember:

Dehydration means shortage of water in the body. It means that a rationing system goes into effect for the available water in the body to determine when, why, and where water should reach various parts of the body. Naturally, the areas that become comparatively dry cannot function normally. These regional or local abnormally functioning areas often produce pain and, eventually, the degenerative disease conditions.

Another way to understand the situation is to compare the effect of dehydration in the body with a shortage of cash flow within the business community in any society. In an economic slump, when the public is not spending money, all business sectors suffer to some extent, some more than others. People cannot go without food, so the producers of food will survive, but not thrive. The housing industry will shrink, the banking industry will suffer from bankruptcies, the car industry will sustain losses, the travel and tourism industry will go broke, and so on.

Another reason why the brain gets priority for water distribution is the *inability* of brain cells to give birth to new daughter cells. They are one-time-living units. If they die, no other cell takes their place. From birth to death, the same cells become educated, cultured, and more and more responsible for controlling the routine functions of the body. To make sure brain cells do not suffer or come to harm, they receive 20 percent of the total circulation, although they constitute only 2 percent of body weight.

Dehydration also causes damage to the liver and its essential manufacturing systems. The liver is the manufacturing and exporting center of many of the most vital elements in the body. It is also the center for detoxification of the chemical by-products of the body. If the liver becomes dehydrated, a number of functions can be lost, some permanently. Likewise, the body's muscles and joints—its locomotive systems—sustain serious damage in dehydration.

For more information about obesity, read my forthcoming book *Obesity: The Deadly Disease of Dehydration.*

CHAPTER 10

DEHYDRATION AND BRAIN DAMAGE

Diseases of the nervous system are so devastating that, unless you have come across people suffering from some of these conditions, you cannot appreciate their devastation. You do not have to be a genius to know that Parkinson's disease, Alzheimer's disease, Lou Gehrig's disease, multiple sclerosis, hemiplegia, quadriplegia, aphasia, autism, attention deficit disorders, and epilepsy, to name some, are dreaded conditions.

I am of the opinion that some of these conditions are produced by persistent dehydration in the body. We need to understand the role of water in the nervous system to realize how easily some of the above problems—those that are not the result of accident or injury, but are gradually establishing degenerative conditions—can be prevented and even cured. An added advantage of preventing brain disease by keeping the brain optimally hydrated is that water increases the brain's efficiency for processing information.

On average, the human brain weighs 1.4 kilograms, or about 3 pounds. It is estimated that the brain consists of 85 percent water, whereas all the other soft-tissue cells are said to be about 75 percent water. The brain is extremely sensitive to water loss. It is said that the brain cannot tolerate even a 1 percent loss of water. If it were to be dehydrated to the point of being only 84 percent water for long, the brain would not function properly. Remember that nerve cells in the brain are one-time-living units. They do not give birth to daughter cells in the same way as other cells in the body. Thus, dehydration that affects a brain cell to the point of causing it damage will leave a permanent mark.

Still, nature is wiser than we think. To make sure that the brain gets all it needs, including all the water, the brain, which is approximately one-fiftieth of the total body weight, is allocated about 20 percent of the circulation. In addition, the brain is constantly bathed in a special fluid composition that is different from blood or serum. The capillaries of the brain manufacture this highly specialized and exact fluid composition. The bulk of these capillaries are inside large chambers of the brain. The fluid they manufacture specially for the brain is called cerebrospinal fluid. It contains more salt and less potassium. This bathing fluid also provides a physically shock-absorbing protection for the brain against knocks to the skull. Also, when the head has to change position rapidly, the fluid surrounding the brain protects it from being thrown about. The brain capillaries also filter and take away the toxic waste produced by the continuously working brain cells. Brain cells function around the clock. The body sleeps, but the brain does not.

THE BLOOD–BRAIN BARRIER

The brain is most effectively protected from fluctuations in the composition of the blood. Unlike the capillaries elsewhere, brain capillaries have no perforations in their walls for the free diffusion of elements. The capillary walls are perfectly sealed. Everything that has to reach the brain side of blood circulation has to be transported by highly specialized and specific mechanisms through the cells lining the capillary wall. You could say the brain capillaries are part of a filter system that regulates the entry of materials into the space that houses the brain itself. In this way, the brain is protected all the time from sudden changes in the composition of the blood. The capillary system of the brain establishes a natural barrier to accessing the brain without a safeguard. This barrier system is called the blood–brain barrier.

Dehydration can cause a breach in the blood–brain barrier. Any such breach compromises the integrity of normal brain functions. I am of the strong opinion that dehydration that compromises the protective shield of the blood–brain barrier is the primary cause of most of the diseases of the central nervous system. When the barrier becomes compromised, the solid waste of such microscopic bleedings is converted into plaques that are the hallmark of most neurological disorders, such as multiple sclerosis, Parkinson's disease, and Alzheimer's disease. I think the same process takes place in migraine headaches.

The same emergency way of hydrating a sensitive area of the body can take place in different organs and tissues. When the system dumps blood into the upper intestine, or if it bleeds into the muscle tissue, 94 percent of the blood volume consists of only water and is immediately put back into circulation. The rationale behind this type of microscopic bleeding in the kidneys and the lungs is that both of these organs need lots of fresh water to begin working properly again. Getting it this way is the only logical process when the body is already dehydrated and no fresh water is coming in to satisfy these organs' needs.

This process of bleeding in the lungs and kidneys, on a microscopic scale, is identified as a distinct condition called pulmonary-renal syndrome. The same process is also seen in lupus, one of the autoimmune diseases. If such bleedings takes place in the intestinal tract on a larger scale and more frequently, the diagnosis of gastritis, duodenitis, or ulcerative colitis is given to the condition. When the process takes place under the skin, particularly in children, it is called a purpura.

In bleeding ulcers, a great deal of blood is dumped into the intestinal tract. Its water is then reabsorbed to avert overconcentration of the blood and the subsequent catastrophic complication of widespread clotting in the brain and elsewhere. I recognized this phenomenon of bleeding in the intestinal tract when I treated more than three thousand cases of peptic ulcer disease with only water. Some of these patients had bleeding ulcers.

I researched the process of bleeding in the intestinal tract some time later and identified the mechanism that I have described. At the time, I treated patients with strongly sweetened water, eight ounces hourly until the bleeding stopped. My reasons for the use of sugar in these cases was the initial assumption that the brain needed a much higher concentration of energy to cope; the secondary reasoning was to switch the mechanism of tissue breakdown to the physiology of tissue formation under the influence of insulin that gets secreted because of sugar. It worked! The bleeding stopped very quickly. Simple water was then used after the bleeding had stopped. This is a treatment process that I recommend in bleeding without a distinct reason. The process of microscopic bleeding into tissues is called *vasculitis*.

NEUROTRANSMITTERS AND DEHYDRATION

Neurotransmitters are brain chemicals that are manufactured and secreted in one or another of the many networks of nerves as a means of passing coded information. The nerve systems in the body are like cables that wire and interconnect the various parts of a country. In the same way that differing codes and wavelengths distinguish one cable television station from another, different chemicals used in the nervous system distinguish the action of one brain center from another. It is interesting to note that up to fifty years ago, scientists had no clear idea as to the mechanism and role of chemical messengers that cause the transfer of information between one nerve and another, or even between the nerve and the muscle fibers it controls and commands.

It is now understood that a number of amino

acids—components of the proteins we eat—are broken down in the cells by specific enzymes, and their by-products become the chemical messengers. The following information is important. Please pay particular attention to the next few paragraphs. I am about to explain why you are a product of what you drink and eat.

We all know that, because of their network of cables to people's homes, telephone companies and cable TV distributors are able to provide other services through their wires, such as Internet and other systems of information and communication that can be connected to computer systems in the house. Their claim to fame is the fact that they have been successful in spreading their wires far and wide. The same wire can be used to pass different coded information all at the same time. All they have to do is to package the information in a particular range of wavelengths of electromagnetic energy. Since we have developed the ability to package information in varying ranges and combination of electrical impulses—wavelengths—that can be transmitted through a cable, we are at a particularly advanced stage in our ability to communicate. Efficient communication and transfer of information between a generating source and users determine the rate of progress and development of any future society. It will make forecasting of events and adoption of an appropriate response possible. The advancement in technology that permits different bundles of information to be transmitted through the same wire at the same time provides a solid foundation for the future progress of society.

The human body has utilized the same technology for the transfer of information in its nerve systems. It has miniaturized the process, and uses chemicals as well as electrical impulses. Nerve cells manufacture one or another brand of chemicals—neurotransmitters—and store them at their nerve endings. Electrical impulses are then passed along the walls of the nerve to where the chemicals are stored and are awaiting release by the electrical trigger system. The electrical impulses travel along the wall of the nerve itself without being shared with the other nerves that are packed in the same bundle. To keep the information private and exclusive to its destination, each nerve has a distinct cylindrical outer layer of insulation that is manufactured mainly from cholesterol—one of cholesterol's many vital and indispensable roles in the body. In most neurological disorders, loss of nerve insulation is a primary contributing factor. It is damage to this insulation layer that causes a variety of symptoms, which are grouped and, in certain circumstances, labeled as "multiple sclerosis."

Another sophistication in the nerve system of the body is the fact that outgoing information is passed in separate nerves to the incoming information that is generated in the rest of the body. The sensations of pain, heat, cold, smell, wetness, sound, light, and sublight ranges of radiation are incoming information. Different chemicals used in the nerve endings identify the central station's main line of function. There are a number of major and minor chemically manipulated nerve systems. However, there are five major groups of nerves that are distinguished by their brand of activity.

They are:
1. *Serotonergic system:* This system uses the serotonin family of chemicals as messengers.
2. *Histaminergic system:* This system uses histamine as a chemical messenger.
3. *Adrenergic system:* This system uses adrenaline, noradrenaline, and dopamine as *their* distinguishing chemical messengers.
4. *Cholinergic system:* This system uses acetylcholine as the chemical messenger.
5. *Opiate system:* This system uses endorphins and enkephalins as the chemical messengers and it is engaged in pain reduction in the body.

These are the biggest and most highly specialized communications corporations in the human body. There seem to be many smaller communications systems that are active, but these function as secondary servers to the main systems.

I would like to mention two of these secondary servers. They employ aspartate and glutamate as their messengers in the brain. I mention these for a purpose. Whereas the other neurotransmitters have to be intricately manufactured and distributed to the nerve endings for their use, aspartate and glutamate do not need to undergo change to register their presence. They act directly on the brain cells that regulate some aspects of the reproductive systems—possibly also growth. Aspar*tate* is a direct by-product of aspar*tame*—the popular artificial sweetener that is used in about five thousand different food products.

Many people who regularly take artificial sweeteners develop a false hunger, and up to ninety minutes after their intake seek food and eat more than they would normally. As a result, they often gain weight. Aspartame may also cause a major disruption in the communications systems of the body with detrimental effects. In certain people with diabetes—a dehydration problem—aspartame has caused diarrhea and intestinal bleeding.

Before it is absorbed, aspartame also produces formaldehyde and methyl alcohol in the intestines. The quantity depends on the amount of sweetener taken in sodas or in cooked food. Formaldehyde and methyl alcohol have been cited as producing eye-nerve damage—to the point of even causing blindness.

Another secondary complication of the use of this sweetener is tumor formation in the brain. Dr. H. J. Roberts of West Palm Beach, Florida, is a dedicated medical doctor who has done much research on the adverse effects of aspartame. He has identified a number of what he calls "aspartame diseases." In his June 2002 article in the *Journal of Townsend Letter for Doctors and Patients*, Dr. Roberts lists a number of neurological problems produced by aspartame. Of twelve hundred patients, 43 percent had headaches; 31 percent had dizziness and unsteadiness; 31 percent had confusion and memory loss; 13 percent had drowsiness and sleepiness; 11 percent had major epileptic convulsions; 3 percent had minor epileptic attacks and "absences of the mind"; 10 percent had severe slurring of speech; 8 percent had tremors; 6 percent had severe "hyperactivity" and "restless legs"; 6 percent had atypical facial pains. He reports that after cutting out the sweetener from the diet of these people, they improved; some were freed of their symptoms. As you might know, methyl alcohol and formaldehyde damage to the brain cells and the optic nerve is irreversible.

SEROTONIN: THE FOREMAN OF ALL NEUROTRANSMITTERS

When tryptophan gets across the blood–brain barrier and reaches the brain side of the divide, it is quickly picked up and converted to a number of neurotransmitters. The best-researched transmitter produced from tryptophan is serotonin, conductor of the orchestra in all brain activity performed by the resident neurotransmitters and master controller of body functions.

A tryptophan by-product that is the rage of the town and the media, because it is available without prescription and is used as a sleeping pill, is melatonin. In the past, tryptophan itself was used in this capacity, before it was taken off the market and the deck was cleared for the introduction of an antidepressant drug called Prozac.

While tryptophan makes more serotonin at a much cheaper cost, Prozac is touted to stop the rapid neutralization of serotonin once it is secreted at the nerve clefts. Why? Because people with depression have low brain-serotonin levels.

Many of the problems in human physiology, and the establishment of stress in the body, are the consequence of the disproportionate transfer of some materials into the brain. In certain circumstances, some amino acids that have to reach the brain cells to be used for making chemical messengers do not reach their destination in sufficient amounts or quickly enough to cope with the demand. The two main causes of shortfall in the delivery of the primary materials are dehydration and the overuse of the respective amino acids in other capacities. Dehydration causes problems with the transport process across the blood–brain barrier.

Tryptophan is vitally important to the human body. It is an essential amino acid. From tryptophan, serotonin, tryptamine, indolamine, and melatonin are manufactured. Tryptophan cannot be manufactured by the body and has to be imported from the foods we eat. This is the reason it is called an essential amino acid. From tyrosine, adrenaline, noradrenaline, and dopamine are manufactured. Six neurotransmitters and one hormone/transmitter—melatonin—become affected when there is dehydration, to the level of producing symptoms such as pain or asthma. The reasons for the loss of these vital elements are simple.

When there is not enough water to detoxify the body through adequate drainage of the tissues and eventually urine production, the liver uses these two amino acids as antioxidants. What are antioxidants? The nearest simple explanation can be seen in the way field lavatories are used without plumbing or drainage. The septic tank of the john contains a chemical that deodorizes, sterilizes, and sanitizes the refuse that gets into the tank when the toilet is used over and over again, until the tank becomes full and has to be emptied by septic pumps. There is a similarity of function between the chemical in the tank and the way the liver uses tryptophan and tyrosine as antioxidants to detoxify the by-products of chemical reactions in the absence of adequate water for washing toxic things out of the body. This is the crudest way of showing how dehydration can cause severe damage to the human brain. It can cause even the brain to malfunction because the raw materials the brain needs become unavailable. From the breakdown of tryptophan, the liver also releases local "oxygen" that is needed for the function of its cells, when the liver is insufficiently supplied!

HISTAMINE: THE FIRST NEUROTRANSMITTER IN OUR BODY

When the sperm fertilizes the female egg and a new living person begins to form, it has the ability to invoke the action of histamine. It must do so because of histamine's many "nursing" responsibilities—it is a wet nurse to growing cells. Histamine will bring the new cells water and nutrients from its direct influence in expanding the blood and serum circulation. Histamine will rhythmically "pump-feed" the new cells with potassium. It is this feeding program that matures the new cell until it divides and divides yet again, and again, until a new life in the form of a fetus comes into being. Histamine is a most noble element in our body.

Histamine also has responsibilities in antibacterial, antiviral, and anti-foreign-agent (chemicals and proteins) defense systems in the body. At a normal level of body-water content, these actions are held at an imperceptive or unexaggerated level. In a dehydrated state of the body, when much histamine is produced, an immune system activation will release an exaggerated amount of the transmitter from histamine-producing cells.

The excess histamine is held in storage for its drought-management program, yet its immune system stimulation will cause a greater-than-required release of the agent. Histamine-producing cells release their histamine reserves, and they immediately begin to divide and create new histamine-producing cells. Now more cells are formed and more histamine is manufactured for its immediate release. This mechanism is designed to cope with emergency water needs or immune system activity. When water comes to an area, it brings with it all the other substances that are also needed. Water is the common factor on which all the regulatory systems are standardized.

It has been shown that in more watery solutions, the histamine-producing cells lose their histamine granules and stop its manufacture for some time. Thus, water seems to be a most effective natural antihistamine. In conditions such as asthma and allergies, excess histamine action is the main problem. These conditions are related and should be regulated with an alert and determined increase in water intake.

The natural anti-asthma and anti-allergic reactions to excess histamine are adrenaline or its chemical substitutes. The natural and preventive procedure to avoid attacks of asthma or allergic reactions is without doubt an adequate hydration of the body over a long period of time. Adequate water intake will reduce the over-production of histamine in the body. A water intake of one or two glasses will cause stimulation of the sympathetic nervous system that secretes adrenaline for at least ninety minutes. This is the main way that water will immediately counteract histamine overactivity. Another solution is to exercise, to again enhance the natural activity of adrenaline in the body. Adrenaline is the natural antidote to excess histamine production.

WATER: THE ENERGIZER OF THE BRAIN

It needs be understood that even if the outer skin of the body is comparatively dry and firm, the inner parts of the body should be waterlogged. All the cells of the body live as though they are in an ocean of salt water. Any function of the body has to obey the natural maritime laws. All transport and communications systems inside and outside the cells of the body are designed based on a water atmosphere, much like the habitat of fish in the ocean.

All functions of the body depend on the basic relationship of its pump systems to water. Imagine people living in rural areas next to a river. Imagine the technology is so advanced that each house has its own small hydroelectric-power-generation system that is installed on the river. The flow of water in the river has the power and ability to turn the waterwheel of the turbines that manufacture electricity for the houses. At present, the turbines made for this type of use are installed separately from their waterwheels. The turbines have to be kept in a dry area, and the electricity they generate is "wired" to the house and distributed. In its use of hydroelectric energy for its cell functions, the human body has advanced beyond human imagination—a most enviable achievement. It has designed special turbines (as it were) that are installed in the waterwheels themselves, and they are submerged deep in the waterways.

Miniaturizing the turbines in this way makes another breakthrough in power generation in the body. As a result of this breakthrough, it has become possible to install each turbine where hydroelectric energy is needed. This makes it possible to economize on the need to use wires or electrical insulation to energize the whole body from its hydroelectric source of energy. The energy-generating battery of turbines is installed where energy is needed to perform a function. These hydroelectric-energy-generating units, which also perform a number of other functions, are called cation (pronounced cat-i-on) pumps.

The human body has made another enviable advancement. Normally, in industrial settings, power is generated in one spot and used in another spot to turn motors that perform particular functions. In the body, the water-dependent, energy-generating components and work-performing functions are installed in the same unit.

To economize further, when the workload is not too excessive and the rate of energy generation is more than is needed, the extra energy is stored. If the rate of water flow is more than adequate, the extra energy that is manufactured is stored in the batteries, like the coal and coke dump reserves next to the power stations that manufacture and distribute electricity. The widely scattered batteries that store the extra energy are called adenosine triphosphate (ATP) and guanosine triphosphate (GTP). A third area where energy is stored is in the calcium dumps in the cells. These areas are known as endoplasmic reticulum.

Imagine a sump or bilge pump in the basement of your house or in a ship that becomes directly energized by the rise in the level of water and is able to generate its own energy from the flow of that water through its system. Now imagine the water is not clear but has other substances floating in it. Please take one further step in the realm of imagination.

Imagine you are a fish living in an intricately designed house in the middle of the ocean, and all of your belongings are afloat. Imagine that you are particularly organized and wish to keep your house spic-and-span and prevent it from getting cluttered up by too many unwanted elements. You would install an automated house-cleaning system—obviously powered by hydroelectricity. The human body has gone through all of these steps in the design of each of its many trillions of cells. It employs a type of "bilge pump," the cation pump.

Cation pumps maintain balance in the interior of the cells of the body. They use hydroelectric energy generated from the rush of water through them to take some elements outside the cell and assist in the transfer of the needed elements into the cell. They energize the cells by also making more power than they need for their own task. This extra energy is stored for later use. Extra energy is manufactured only when water supply and its pressure is adequate. All functions of the brain depend in a major way on this source of energy.

It is my understanding that the microtubules in the waterways of all cells, including the long nerves, are made of cation pumps that are stuck together. You now understand why the rush of water from the outside to the inside of the microtubules also turns all the energy-dependent cation pumps that make up the microtubule.

Next to oxygen, water is the most essential material for the efficient working of the brain. Water is a primary nutrient for all brain functions and transmission of information. This is why the brain is 85 percent water and is housed in a very special "water bag" that goes all the way down the spinal cord into the lower back. The use of cation pumps is not limited to the nervous system. They are employed in all the cells of the body, in their outer membranes and in the membranes inside the cells.

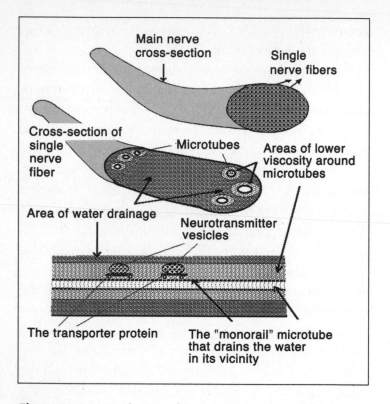

Figure 10.1: A single axon that is cut across shows the micro-tubules and the areas of more fluidity that seem to allow the existence of a "float"-transport system along the line of the tube.

A few years ago, I received a letter from a woman who is worth mentioning here. She wrote about an ear problem that is now cleared up. The story exemplifies my explanations of chronic dehydration and nerve damage. She was a young-at-heart, seventy-one-year-old professional concert musician who taught at her local university. She was very health-conscious, ate the right kind of foods, but drank green tea and only two cups of water a day, and did not take salt. She did exercise. One day she realized her left ear could not hear properly and had lost the ability to distinguish fine sounds. She went for ear tests at two different centers. Both reached the conclusion that she was suffering from some nerve deafness, which was not advanced enough to warrant her wearing a hearing aid. She wondered about acupuncture treatment and had six sessions of it, "but it didn't help." Then she heard me on a radio interview explaining chronic dehydration as a major cause of so many health problems. She bought my book *Your Body's Many Cries for Water* and, after reading it, began drinking more water. The result: "After about a month I found I could and still can hear the watch tick with my left ear." This simple observation on "nerve recovery" by a person who was alert to the loss of an important function is an indication of how chronic dehydration can lead to devastating results, and how correction of dehydration in time can reverse a potentially permanent pathology.

DEHYDRATION: THE CAUSE OF STROKES

Talking about permanent pathology, let me tell you the story of my sister Shahla. We are a close family, and there is a particular bond between my sister and me. There is about thirteen years' difference between us. When we were studying in England, away from home and parents, I was in charge. Even in later stages of her life, whenever she needed to make a serious decision, she would consult with me. As a family, we emigrated to America when living in our homeland, Iran, became hazardous after the mullahs took over in 1979 and Iran became a theocratic dictatorship. Most of us gravitated to northern Virginia.

Shahla is a hard worker and a most reliable executive, and although she had a lot of upheaval in her life in exile she has not lost her cheerfulness and enthusiasm. She had recently started smoking despite my contrary advice. She had also taken a liking to a glass of red wine now and then. She had come to Virginia to work with my younger brother, who had established himself as a developer in the area.

In the summer of 1989, Shahla wanted to relax after a lot of turmoil in her emotional life. She decided to spend some time beside the pool of her apartment complex. She was also trying to lose weight. She would spend most of her free time and the weekends at the poolside in the sun. She would also take the occasional drink of wine as she was relaxing on her poolside mat—an ideal of many people who wish to have a quiet, relaxing holiday.

On a Monday morning after a weekend by the pool, when she was working at her office, she noticed tingling sensations in her left arm. Gradually the left side of her body became heavy and not sufficiently responsive. She got scared and called me. She left the office and was driven home. By the time I arrived, her left leg and left arm were in a state of partial paralysis. She could hardly move them. She was now dead scared. After a quick examination and a call to a doctor

friend, I started to force water into her. I managed to
give her two jugs of water and one jug of orange juice
with some salt, about six quarts of fluids. Her anxiety
began to diminish. By the time the doctor had arrived,
her arm weakness had perceptibly improved and she
also had some movement in her leg muscles.

You might think that I should have called an ambu-
lance and packed her off to the emergency room of a
hospital. I did not do so because, other than receiving
an intravenous drip to get some fluid into her, I
believe she would have suffered other damage in the
time she awaited medical attention. Anyway, she
improved and improved and improved. By the late
afternoon, she was well on her way to recovery. However, we needed to find out if there was any underlying
local pathology in the brain that might have signaled
its presence by manifesting muscle weakness on one
side of her body.

A consultation with one of the local neurologists
was arranged, and we went to him for an in-depth
evaluation. After his examination, he confirmed a
slight remaining weakness on the left side. Shahla was
admitted to the hospital. After all the blood tests and
noninvasive procedures such as CT scans and MRIs
showed nothing, it was decided to do a cerebral
angiogram to rule out a leaking aneurysm in the brain
arteries.

The procedure was conducted the next day. Her
brain arteries were as clean as a whistle. No aneurysm,
no plaque, no obstruction, nothing that would
account for the temporary weakness on the left side of
her body. They charged her thirteen thousand dollars

for three nights' stay in the hospital. She did not yet have insurance to cover such expenses. Needless to say, what rest she had at the poolside she paid for with her health and money. Why? Because of a basically wrong understanding of the way the human body works.

She had severely dehydrated her brain by the intake of alcohol, heat of the sun, dieting without water intake, and the vicious cycle of the physiological events that are set in motion when there is severe dehydration. What her brain had done was to decommission a major part of its activity that would take her to the location where she could continue the damage-producing actions.

Even in genuine situations when there is a blockage of the arteries in a region of the brain, resulting in "rotting" brain tissue, adequate intravenous hydration has produced dramatic recoveries. In experiments in animals, if intravenous fluids are given within one hour of blocking the main artery to a part of the brain that would permanently destroy about 20 percent of the blood-deprived region, the rotting area will be reduced significantly. Such is the power of water in reviving even purposely oxygen- and circulation-deprived areas of the brain.

This was the reason why I forced water on Shahla as soon as I reached her. I thought that even if she had actually clotted one of the main arteries of her brain, the water would help open the surrounding capillaries and prevent expansion of the clot beyond its already formed areas. Equally, if the neurological manifestations were due to vascular spasm, then the water would relieve the constriction in the arteries—and it did. There was no time to wait and see; a decision and an action were vital at the very moment that Shahla showed the onset of muscle weakness that was increasing. Today, she is well. She no longer smokes, and drinks wine only on festive occasions, but drinks plenty of water—enough to give her lots of bubbly energy.

Edmund, the husband of my office manager, a very young man, had exactly the same type of paralysis and was taken to the hospital. His wife, Joy, was informed of the devastating crisis in their family. I was nearby when she received the information. I asked her if Edmund drank enough water. Apparently he would seldom drink water. I asked her to get him to drink lots of water straightaway to prevent the damage from continuing. She did, and he recovered completely. It is now four years since that episode.

The moral of these stories: Give stroke candidates lots of water—if possible, before they actually develop clots and then neurological symptoms.

CHAPTER 11

HORMONES AND DEHYDRATION

Stress to the human body immediately translates into dehydration. In other words, stress equals dehydration, and dehydration equals stress. They both initiate the same series of physiological steps for crisis management. Immediate and automatic steps are taken to prepare the body for "battle stations." The available body resources of water and food products will be distributed according to battle-station requirements. How is this done? Five major regulators become operatives of the system. These regulators have their individual codes, which are indicators of one or another mode of activity through their cascade of chemical reactions, much like the directives of a central command that are delivered to the commanders in the field.

Vasopressin

Vasopressin indicates a water shortage and a rationing of water delivery into the interior of certain cells according to a priority plan. It opens small holes in the cell membrane and forces water through the membrane so that cells sensitive to vasopressin will benefit more from the available water supply. This allows the brain, kidneys, liver, and other organs to maintain efficiency, particularly when the blood becomes more concentrated from the breakdown of muscle and fat. Vasopressin regulates water delivery into the cells until there is an unmistakable signal of abundant water supply for all body functions. Vasopressin also tightens the arterial system to put a squeeze on the blood volume to force serum out of the vessels. This enables some of the water content of the serum to enter the dehydrated cells through the holes in their membrane.

Once vasopressin becomes secreted, it acts as a strong on–off–on (modulating) stimulant for the release of cortisone. It is a very strong cortisone release factor. It is this action of vasopressin that converts persistent dehydration into a metabolic problem that can cause serious disruption in the reserves of the body's essential elements (see figure 7.4).

Cortisone Release Factor

Cortisone release factor promotes the secretion of hormones from the adrenal glands, which rest on top of the kidneys. Cortisone promotes the breakdown of proteins, fats, and stored starch into their primary components, some of which will be converted to sugar for brain use. This process will eventually deplete some of the essential amino acids, such as tryptophan and tyrosine, from the stored reserves of the body. As a result, many health problems that are the consequence of prolonged dehydration may develop. Cortisone directly suppresses the body's immune system. It is this mechanism that results in immune system suppression when the body becomes dehydrated and remains dehydrated. Production of interferon and interleukin-2—the vital activators of the immune system—is inhibited by cortisone.

The lost essential elements are not easily replaceable. The body can become short of some of its most essential amino acid needs for protein manufacture. Some of this loss can become irreversible. Even if raw materials are made available at a later time, the same state of physiology as before may not be attainable. Thus, muscle activity to avert the damaging effect of stress is indispensable—hence the need to walk, walk, and walk. Increased water intake to avert the physiological damage of stress is even more important.

Endorphins

These are the natural opiates of the body. They bring about immediate pain relief at the time of battle; they enhance the efficiency of the body in the process of fight or flight. When the body is exposed to injury or great stress, endorphins are released. Bleeding and severe pain also promote endorphin release. Endorphins raise the pain threshold so the body is able to endure and effectively continue to function to the last moment, despite physical trauma. Long-distance runners become dependent on the release of endorphins to continue until completion of a marathon race. When there is no injury or trauma, endorphin release translates to well-being and gratification.

Women often have a much greater dependence on the endorphin codes for their pain relief, especially for the physically traumatic processes of pregnancy and childbirth. Generation after generation of women have passed this strong ability for the expression of endorphin code to their offspring. It has become a stronger part of the chromosome code for the female of all species, particularly humans. This is why women have a greater ability to endure pain than men, and also why they live longer.

Alcohol is a dehydrating agent. Furthermore, it inhibits the full and widespread actions of vasopressin, causing further dehydration. In women, alcohol initiates release of endorphins. The more alcohol that is consumed, the more endorphin high will be experienced as a consequence of cellular dehydration. The addictive property of alcohol is most probably the consequence of endorphin release from the process of establishing dehydration. Although the process is the same in men and women, in women it becomes more strongly and rapidly addictive than in men. The reason lies in the women's ability to activate more quickly the endorphin-manufacturing system and its release in alcohol-induced stress. This is probably why women become addicted to alcohol in about two to three years, whereas men become addicted in about seven years.

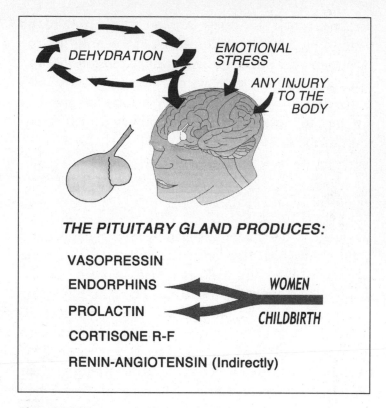

Figure 11.1

Renin-Angiotensin (RA)

The RA system codes for water intake and its retention and distribution in the body by forcing a salt
appetite and the collection of salt in the watery areas
outside the cells. It is responsible for closing some of
the blood vessels in the periphery so that the shunting
of circulation to other more vital parts, according to a
priority plan, can be established. It is also responsible
for decreased urine production. It is produced in the

kidneys, which play a part in water preservation of the body. The RA system is a focus of attention by the pharmaceutical industry in antihypertension therapy. Instead of giving the system more water to pass through the kidneys, chemical products are given to attempt to block the drive of the body for salt retention by the RA system.

Prolactin

Prolactin codes for breast-gland-cell stimulation and milk production. It coordinates with other hormone agents to maintain the reproductive organs of the body in a well-functioning state. The milk-producing tissue is a water-secreting gland, and its milk-water-secretory capability has to be maintained. Gland cells have to be activated and given secretory properties. If such cells are already formed and functioning, their activity has to be maintained. At times of stress, when the water-rationing system becomes operative, breast function has to be maintained to feed the offspring of the species. In a very severe state of stress, this milk-secretion property of prolactin may not be enough, and milk production may have to stop. There is a balancing mechanism involved.

In chronic dehydration, or ongoing low-grade stress, there may be a constant and ongoing effect on the breast tissue caused by the increasing amounts of stress-induced prolactin production. If the breast is already fully developed and has had past experience of milk production, the result may be an enlargement of the gland tissue. If the breast tissue is uninitiated, or a long time has elapsed between its initial milk-secretory learning period and the advent of stress, the result of stress-induced increased prolactin production may be cystic adenoma formation. Over a longer period of time, the end result of stress/dehydration-induced increases in prolactin production may be cancer transformation of the adenoma tissue. By this time, because of other damaging effects of dehydration and protein loss, many other controlling and anti-cancer-cell defense systems are already out of commission. The immune system is suppressed, and interferon production is decreased as a result of too much cortisone release. I am of the opinion that cancer of the breast in the majority of women is the consequence of chronic dehydration, associated with stress.

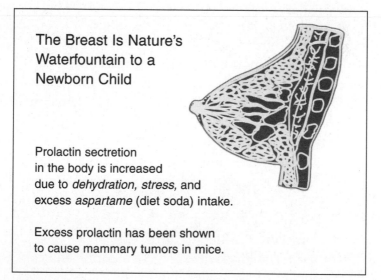

The Breast Is Nature's
Waterfountain to a
Newborn Child

Prolactin sectretion
in the body is increased
due to *dehydration, stress,* and
excess *aspartame* (diet soda) intake.

Excess prolactin has been shown
to cause mammary tumors in mice.

Figure 11.2

DEPRESSION AND CHRONIC FATIGUE SYNDROME

As mentioned, the brain uses a great deal of electrical energy that is manufactured by the water drive of the energy-generating pumps. With dehydration, the level of energy generation in the brain is decreased. The ATP pool of energy becomes gradually depleted, more at some sites of activity than others. Many silent functions of the brain that depend on hydroelectric energy become inefficient. We recognize this inadequacy of function and call it depression.

To the human body, caffeine is very much like the booster system in an engine. In the same way a booster system burns fuel at a faster but inefficient rate to propel a car or plane at an exaggerated speed, so caffeine forces an increase in consumption of ATP. Caffeine in coffee, tea, and other beverages forces an excess expenditure of ATP energy by the brain. The brain always keeps some energy in reserve for emergency use—such as the energy surge of the last few miles of a marathon runner. Caffeine also dehydrates the body. One cup of coffee or tea, or a glass of an alcoholic drink, produces more urine than the actual ingested volume of liquid of any of the beverages. On top of that, by trying to cool down the body temperature to adjust for the hot tea or coffee, more water is lost in the form of perspiration. Tea addicts are always thirsty, but they continue to drink tea.

Normally, low levels of ATP give a lasting and constant signal of a lowered level of energy. This signal of a low battery reading puts the system on guard and does not permit the overuse of the ATP energy pool in the cell. In this way, each cell will have a fatigue signal of its own. It will take far stronger stimulus than before to fire up these fatigued cells. Consequently, the conscious mind is deprived of the possibility of accessing the cells' ATP energy pool, and will function at a less efficient level. Even the volition to perform a function is lost. It should be remembered that there is a time gap between energy expenditure from the ATP pool and the remanufacture of the spent energy, so the brain will operate at less-than-normal efficiency or at a depressed level for some time.

It seems that caffeine and other chemical stimulants alter the level at which spent ATP registers its signals of lower battery reading. Eventually, these stimulants may not be able to overcome the inhibitory influence of ATP loss. There may even come a time when *almost* no ATP is left to tap into for outside work. Now all a cell can do is stop most of its functions in order to survive. More and more, the body loses its ability to use brain energy to do mental or physical work, and the person becomes passive, in a vegetative mode of social behavior. What began as a depression now becomes a generalized fatigue. Once you add the problems of chronic dehydration to mental fatigue, a conglomerate of many different symptom-producing states with a general label of "chronic fatigue syndrome" (CFS) is born.

CFS is a manufactured label to describe a series of disparate symptoms and signs. In different parts of the world, the same series of conditions are labeled "postviral fatigue syndrome," "neuromyasthenia," "myalgic neuroencephalomyelitis"—tongue-twisting labels that mean little. Until it was shown to be an inaccurate assumption, it was thought that CFS was caused by the Epstein-Barr virus.

There is a clear relationship between the stresses associated with lifestyle trends that result in an upheaval in the metabolic and physiological balance of the body and the condition known as CFS. For those persons who have a strong leaning toward the belief that CFS is a viral disease, I recommend reading the section on lupus in my book *ABC of Asthma, Allergies and Lupus*. I describe how initial dehydration is responsible for fragmentation of the DNA of some cells into small particles that have been classified as viruses (see figure 7.4).

We should never forget that the body is a conglomerate of chemical systems. It is able to build new tissue, or break up already formed structures, as a means of recycling the raw materials. Other than the brain, no part of the body is sacrosanct—even muscle tissue is broken down to tap into its stored amino acid pool. In continuous stressful encounters and life patterns, this is exactly what happens, whether the stress is caused by an emotional experience or by fighting a viral infection. *Dehydration, stress, and dieting for aesthetic value, without the benefits of exercise,* in my opinion, must be assumed to be the root causes of CFS, particularly if pick-me-up fluids such as coffee or alcohol are taken as substitutes for the water needs of the body.

One of the major needs of the body is salt. In dehydration and dieting that excludes salt intake, the body will become salt-depleted. Salt is essential for muscle and nerve activity. In hot climates, when too much sweating causes salt deficiency, one of the symptoms often seen is a lack of energy to undertake any form of activity. Another symptom is muscle aches and cramps. Persons suffering from CFS should test increasing their salt intake at the same time as they increase their water intake—naturally, with total exclusion of caffeine-containing pick-me-ups. They have to allow some time for the buildup of their ATP reserves and full recovery of the delivery systems in the nerve fibers.

DRY AND BURNING EYES

Tear production for the normal functions of the eye is absolutely essential. In some people, this function is deficient and the eyes feel a burning sensation. Much blinking may take place to promote circulation to the tear glands. If this is ineffective, the eyes will be forced to shut to prevent water loss by evaporation. In some people, like myself, who may have had Bell's palsy (an obstruction of the facial nerve that also causes paralysis of the face muscles on that side), tear formation in one eye often becomes affected. The eye on the side of the paralysis will become drier than the other, even when the muscles have partially recovered. It is my personal experience that even if rubbing the eye does not promote tear formation and wetting of the eye, two glasses of water alleviates the condition fairly promptly. The burning and pain should disappear in minutes. Artificial tears or frequent washing of the face and letting water get into the eyes will also help.

HIGHER BLOOD CHOLESTEROL

Everyone is now conscious of raised cholesterol as a marker of potential diseases of the heart and brain— the consequences of clogged arteries. In 1987, at an international gathering of cancer research scientists in Greece, I exposed the scientific reasons why increased cholesterol production in the body is a direct consequence of chronic dehydration.

We have to assume that the genetic structure of each cell empowers it to act independently, if environmental conditions are not to its advantage. The cells of the human body have the same capability as bacteria to adapt to their environment by altering their membrane structure. Similarly, human body cells alter the cholesterol content of their membranes to prevent the uncontrolled seepage of water in or out of their inner domains. Normally, water is meant to seep into the cell at a slow but exact rate.

Cells also possess a mechanism for getting rid of excess water. However, if the cell water has to be kept inside because its environment is becoming comparatively dry, the cell membrane has to be sealed off. Cholesterol deposits within the structure of the membrane carry out the process of sealing off the membrane—the very pores that allow water to diffuse through get sealed off.

Normally, when food is eaten, water and enzymes

have to be poured into the stomach and intestines. The enzymes break the food particles into their smaller building blocks by inserting one molecule of water at each of the amino acids' many points of bondage that make up the protein structure and mass. Free water is used up to allow this action to take place. The result is that the body has less water and more soluble solid matter that needs to be transported in the now comparatively water-depleted blood and lymph circulation.

The result of this digestive process is concentrated blood that leaves the intestines and goes through the liver. In the liver, some of this food load is taken away from the blood, and the balance is poured into the heart at the right side. At this right heart entrance, the lymph from the intestine also pours into the blood. The first place that this concentrated and now circulating blood visits is the lung tissue. Here more water in the form of vapor is lost from the circulating blood during the breathing process.

Now this concentrated blood is brought to the left side of the heart and pumped out. It goes to the arteries that feed the heart itself, then to the arteries of the brain, and then to the main body artery, called the aorta. When this concentrated blood reaches the brain centers that deal with the osmotic regulation of the body, they signal the conscious mind that the body is short of water. The alarm for thirst develops, and the person feels the urge to drink water.

There is a fairly long time gap between the exposure of the liver cells and the cell lining of the arteries to the concentrated blood and the time water is taken into the body. The time gap of water intake after food and the dehydrating influence of concentrated blood is sufficient to cause a cholesterol-amassing and generating activity in those cells that come in contact with the concentrated blood—such as the liver and the lining of the arteries. In time, a physiological pathway for the manufacture and deposit of cholesterol in the lining of the blood vessels will occur. The only way the cells that cannot form cholesterol can protect themselves is to pick up cholesterol from the circulation and deposit it in their membranes.

Raised cholesterol is a sign that the cells of the body have developed a defense mechanism against the stronger osmotic forces of blood. The concentrated blood would normally keep drawing water out through the cell membranes. Cholesterol is a natural sort of waterproof clay that, when poured in the gaps of the cell membrane, helps keep the membrane's architecture intact and prevents excess water loss. In chronic dehydration, additional amounts of cholesterol will continue to be produced by the liver cells and poured into the circulation for the common use of all cells that do not possess the power to manufacture their own. The additional cholesterol will also make the cell wall impervious to the passage of water that naturally takes place in a normally well-hydrated cell.

To prevent excess cholesterol deposits by the cells lining the arteries and the liver, you need to drink regularly an ample amount of water a half hour before food intake. By this action, the cells of the body will become well hydrated before confronting the concentrated blood after food intake. There will also be enough water for the processes of digestion and respiration, without needing to tap into the water held inside the cells lining the blood vessels.

After a period of regulating daily water intake so that the cells gradually become fully hydrated, the cholesterol defense system will be required less, and its production will decrease. In light of this information, the range of normal blood cholesterol will probably prove to be far less than the values quoted at present. It is now becoming apparent that effective reduction of cholesterol levels in the circulating blood could promote a clearing of already formed deposits.

I had occasion to advise a man in his early forties whose angiogram had revealed partial blockage of his coronary arteries. The blockage was such that he had developed chest pains. I advised him not to have bypass surgery without first trying a conservative treatment for his condition. He agreed to adjust his daily water intake and to begin by taking two glasses (just under one pint) of water exactly half an hour before each meal. I advised him to walk one hour in the morning and one hour in the evening (to start with, twenty to thirty minutes at the beginning, increasing gradually to one hour).

I explained that research has shown that the hormone-sensitive, fat-digesting enzymes become activated after the first hour of walking, and remain active for twelve hours. The reason for the twice-daily walk was the need to activate the fat-burning enzyme on a regular basis and for its recognized cumulative action. Three months later the man went to one of the famous centers in Houston for a final checkup and an assessment of his need for bypass surgery His new angiogram showed no sign of the previous blockage He no longer needed surgery.

CORONARY HEART DISEASE

The basics of this condition are explained in the above section on cholesterol formation and its deposit in the coronary arteries. Not much more can be added on this topic. If we also take into consideration that another basic cause of diseases of the heart is continued hypertension and the shearing force of concentrated circulating blood, then the application of the same information will explain the root cause of coronary heart disease and brain damage and strokes.

It should be remembered that this information applies to all cells in each organ. When there is dehydration, all cells in all organs feel the problem, except some feel it more than others, until an emergency water-infusion system begins to hydrate the more essential cells. The heart is not exempt from the problems associated with dehydration. It becomes sufficiently incapacitated to begin showing failure. Often the process begins with the spasm, and then permanent obstruction, of a small artery. The initial spasm causes pain. If at that very moment water is taken, the spasm will subside and the permanent obstruction of the artery may not be the outcome. In any case, water is immediately more essential to the patient than any other medication. It will at least reduce the extent of the damage. High blood cholesterol can also be an indicator of bone density loss. For more information, read the sections Higher Blood Cholesterol and Osteoporosis.

HOT FLASHES

As I have explained, the nerve sensors of the face receive the same attention for their circulation as do the cells of the brain because they are directly involved with information gathering. At their brain side, they are connected to the serotonin-regulated nerve system that, at the same time, has a regulatory role in the hormonal balance of the body. The level of tryptophan and serotonin activity in the body is directly influenced by the regulatory role of water.

Because of the age-dependent loss of thirst sensation and the establishment of persistent dehydration, at some point or other in the life of any individual, the hormonal balance of the body will automatically become affected by the same dehydration. In women, this hormonal imbalance will eventually lead to symptom-producing menopause and its hallmark of hot flashes. Historically, some women are known for having given birth to a child when they were in their seventies. It is therefore feasible that there is no hard-and-fast rule to the age in which menopause is established. With the right lifestyle and balanced nutrition, it may be possible to delay menopause and alleviate its symptoms.

To treat hot flashes, you need to hydrate the body well. You need to take a balanced amino acid diet that enhances the serotonin activity of the brain. You also need to take vitamin B_6 as a supplement. Vitamin B_6 is directly involved in the conversion of the amino acids: tryptophan to serotonin, melatonin, tryptamine, and indolamine; tyrosine to dopa, dopamine, noradrenaline, and adrenaline; histidine to histamine. These neurotransmitters are vital for balancing the hormonal functions of the body, as well as its water-intake regulation. Dehydrated people are all vitamin B_6–and zinc-deficient. The addition of 100 milligrams of B_6 to your daily diet will prevent hot flashes and alleviate PMS. This prudent precaution will also correct a range of other problems too extensive to discuss here.

GOUT

When the body begins to collect uric acid, and this substance is seen in some of the joints of the body at the same time as there is joint pain, this condition is called gout. Uric acid is a product of incomplete protein metabolism. It seems to be associated with the advanced complications of dehydration. It has been my clinical experience that increased water intake to the point that the urine is always free of color will avert attacks of gout pain. It is my view that formation of uric acid crystals and their collection in the joints is a direct result of chronic dehydration.

KIDNEY STONES

Inadequate water intake and urine concentration are assumed to be responsible for the formation of uric acid and calcium deposits in the renal tissue. Once a primary crystal of these elements has formed, new deposits are made and larger pieces develop until they can become large enough to cause obstruction. Urinary infection will promote stone formation. If kidney stones are formed and passed, realize that you are suffering from a long-term effect of dehydration. The urine should never have become so concentrated as to cause the formation of the initial crystal seeds, which can grow into large stones within the kidneys.

SKIN AND DEHYDRATION

In a dehydrated state of the body, the first site for establishing water conservation is the skin. Skin has the ability to perspire or sweat to cool and regulate body temperature. If there is dehydration, the water reserves in the skin may be used up without being replaced at the same rate as the water is lost. Thus, dehydration is a primary factor in the production of dry and lusterless skin: One, the skin loses moisture and becomes dry and prunelike; two, there is less capillary circulation to the skin area to give it the healthy color it should have. To promote a healthier skin, adequate water intake is essential.

Human skin is the tissue that houses the inner workings of the body. Its cells need water all the time.

They are exposed to the environment and lose water through surface evaporation, perspiration, and sweating—three different rates of water loss from the skin surface. If water does not reach the skin from the circulation at its base, the rate of skin repair will decrease, and dehydrated cells will cover the body.

This is one of the reasons why you often see young women with their skins already aged beyond their years; why you see middle-aged women with deep furrows—crow's feet—all over their faces. The face is most exposed to wind and the sun's rays, elements that enhance water loss from the skin's surface. Men have coarser skin than women, which is why men's skin does not show its damage from dehydration as readily as women's skin. Men have another advantage. In order to make facial hair grow, male hormones bring more circulation to the skin of the face. Nonetheless, persistent dehydration does produce rough and furrowed skin in men's faces, too.

The ultimate in dehydration-produced skin problems is scleroderma—the skin becomes atrophied and thin, or scaly like an alligator's hide. In its early stages of scleroderma, the skin begins to resemble a crocodile's. Exposed areas of the skin—arms, knees, shins, hands, and feet—are first to show the sign of the disease. The skin becomes fibrous, thick, and scaly. At later stages the skin becomes very thin and almost "shrink-wraps" the anatomical parts under it. When it affects the face, it can disfigure the nose, mouth, and eyes, as if the person is wearing a pale, shiny mask. The condition is very painful as well.

The good news is that at its early phase, scleroderma can be reversed by increased water intake. I have seen the change back to normal skin in a young woman who was ecstatic with the outcome. She had been dreading the progress of her seemingly incurable crippling problem. What amazes me is the number of ways the human body can manifest dehydration—and how we in medicine have never understood the missing role of water in the conditions we have labeled diseases.

The most common irritant to the skin is the detergent residue on washed clothes that are not well rinsed. The detergent can dissolve in sweat and cause contact dermatitis and even hives. Always double rinse anything you wash.

OSTEOPOROSIS

Osteoporosis is normally recognized in the sixth decade of life, although it often starts in the body fifteen to twenty years earlier. It occurs in both sexes and in all population groups. The total bone mass seems to decrease. It seems that the rate of bone resorption exceeds the rate of bone formation. Consequently, bone consistency and volume begin to decline. No one knows why osteoporosis occurs as we age. What I am about to discuss is my view. It is new and not necessarily subscribed to by others in the field of scientific research.

By linking osteoporosis to chronic dehydration and a gradual rise in cholesterol levels of the body, I am sure I will incur the wrath of many of my colleagues who are looking at the condition through solutes-directed research. Be that as it may, the following is my scientific belief and worthy of being exposed. Should my views prevail, the solution to osteoporosis will become simple. It will be a matter of *prevention*, nine-tenths of any sensible cure. To expose the relationship between osteoporosis and dehydration, we need to understand how bone formation takes place in the human body.

As an example, and depending on the availability of raw materials at a construction site, the use of concrete for the building of the skeleton of a building seems to be the most practical, long-lasting, and economical method. If sand, gravel, and cement are locally produced, water is the only other necessary element to mix these components and the interwoven steel rods, which act as internal trusses for the cement to hold on to, as well as providing the rigidity needed for any durable building construction. Exactly the same principle is employed in the manufacture of skeletal bones.

The architecture of dense bones employs myriad interwoven collagen fibers. Single fibers are anchored together and woven into a three-ply band. The woven bands are laid side by side and anchored together. It seems these thicker ropelike structures are now interwoven in such a way that "hole zones" or gaps are created for the deposit of a number of different calcium and sodium crystals. While the elastic collagen fibers provide the inner scaffolding for the calcium, the calcium itself establishes the necessary rigidity for the bone to become weight-bearing. Also, much of the 24 percent deposit of sodium in the body—along with the other minerals, such as magnesium, that are not dissolved in extracellular fluid—is stored as crystals in the bone. Thus, bone formation depends on calcium, sodium, and, to a lesser degree, other mineral deposits.

Now that we are discussing sodium, let us recognize an important fact. Sodium and its "attached" chloride or bicarbonate constitute 90 percent of all the solids dissolved in the fluid surrounding the cells of the body. Thus, sodium is the most important ingredient for the maintenance of extracellular fluid volume. Twenty-four percent of all the sodium in the body seems to be in a solid and crystalline form, mainly stored in the bones. The stored sodium in the bone must be assumed to compose the sodium reserves of the body, at the same time as it is employed for bone crystallization and rendering it hard. Thus, sodium in its own right serves an important function in the process of bone formation. Sodium shortage in the body, now that we understand its role in bone formation, may be a contributing factor in the establishment of osteoporosis. A sodium-free diet and the long-term use of diuretics may be a contributory factor in the establishment of osteoporosis.

Collagen fibers are manufactured from amino acids that are connected in a linear fashion. The amino acid pool of the body seems to regulate the manufacture of these fibers. These fibrous strands are protected from being enzymatically broken if they are deeply embedded in the calcium deposits. As soon as the calcium is removed from around the fibers, their enzymatic breakdown and the reentry of their amino acid components into the amino acid pool becomes possible. This is how bone formation of the body has to do a balancing act between bone construction and bone breakdown. A tip of balance in the direction of one or the other state determines whether bone becomes thicker and more solid, or weak and lighter in construction.

How does bone resorption takes place? How is it related to dehydration?

There are many different factors involved in bringing about bone resorption to the point of causing osteoporosis. I will not get involved in the variety of conditions that have bone resorption as their indirect consequence. I will concentrate on the possible direct relationship of dehydration to osteoporosis. Remember that there is normally a time gap between the exposure of a disease process and the initiating factors that began the process. In the case of the onset of chronic dehydration and its consequence of osteoporosis, my opinion is there may be a gap of one to three decades.

It is my understanding that the very gradual loss of thirst sensation—the primary cause for the establishment of chronic dehydration—begins after the third decade of life, while the establishment of osteoporosis is mostly seen during the sixth decade of life. Thus, the tip of balance in favor of gradual and incipient bone resorption becomes established over the span of many years. Inactivity and disuse of the bone structure accentuate the rate of osteoporosis, while physical activity and the full use of the bones favor the laying down of calcium deposits and strengthening the frame of the bones.

One of the main factors for the establishment of osteoporosis is the process of bone breakdown—osteolysis—that is brought about by prostaglandin E (PGE). As we know, PGE is a subordinate that routinely becomes active at the command of the neurotransmitter histamine. Bone marrow has an abundance of mast cells that manufacture histamine.

The consequence of the prolonged activation of PGE by histamine is tapping into the calcium reserves by means of the breakdown of bone (osteolysis) and the removal of calcium from the bone deposits. The removal of calcium exposes the collagen for ultimate breakdown. In this way, dehydration that commissions histamine into activity will produce the consequent osteoporosis in the bone structures of the body. Osteoporosis is the negative outcome between the rate of bone formation and osteolysis.

The only way to decommission histamine and prevent the bone resorption that is associated with dehydration is to adequately increase daily water intake to no less than eight glasses of water, eight ounces each. You also need sufficient exercise to tip the balance in favor of bone formation. Exercise has many other beneficial effects, of course. Not only does it cause strengthening of the bone itself, as well as its joints and its muscle connections, but it also promotes better circulation—it opens and creates a more extensive capillary bed and builds a larger blood pool to draw on when the body is in need of more water and raw materials. This is why well-exercised people are able to endure hardship and stress with fewer detrimental effects. An adequate and balanced protein diet is also essential to maintain the amino acid pool that ultimately determines the rate of manufacture of different collagen fibers.

CANCER FORMATION

In September 1987, I was asked to deliver the guest lecture at a select cancer conference and workshop, because I had introduced a new understanding to this major health problem of our society. I scientifically explained why chronic unintentional dehydration is, in my view, the primary cause of pain and disease in the human body, including cancer. I explained that dehydration produces a drastic system disturbance in the physiology of the body and causes four major disruptions that ultimately and collectively allow for cancer formation and the invasive growth of the new tissue. My lecture was published in the September–October 1987 issue of the *Journal of Anticancer Research*. You can retrieve this article from my Web site www.watercure.com. Further scientific information is available in my article "Neurotransmitter Histamine: An Alternative Viewpoint," which was presented at the Third Interscience World Conference on Inflammation in 1989. In September 2002, I was invited for the second time to highlight my understanding of dehydration and cancer formation in the body at the Thirty-first Annual Cancer Control Society Conference in Los Angeles.

The detailed explanations are too complicated for the scope of this book, but the highlights are as follows:

Persistent dehydration causes a multisystem dysfunction in the entire physiology of the body, including:

1. DNA damage in the cell nucleus
2. Inefficiency and eventual loss of DNA repair system inside the cells
3. Cell receptor abnormalities and loss of balancing processes of the hormonal control systems
4. General immune system suppression, even at the level of the bone marrow, causing lack of ability to recognize abnormal cells, the inability to destroy them, and loss of the filter system for removal of abnormal and primitive genes from the time-refined and sophisticated gene pool in the body.

In short, dehydration will gradually cause the body to lose its edge against the disruptive cascade of chemical combinations that constitute makeshift processes until the body gets back to its normal pattern of chemistry. You see, the body is a chemical refinery; it is the outcome of a most sophisticated pattern of chemical reactions that depend on the adequate presence of water and, naturally, other food-contained ingredients. If you shortchange it the water it needs to maintain efficiency and run the myriad chemical formulas every second of every minute of life, you cause the creation of new chemical pathways that produce pain, disease, and premature death. Cancer formation is the outcome of a series of such chemical formulas and pathways to early death. Four of these primary pathways have been mentioned above.

The relationship of dehydration and DNA damage is easy to understand. Every cell has the tendency to produce some highly acidic by-products from its chemical reactions. Water has the job of washing these acidic elements out of the cell and taking them to the liver and the kidneys to be processed. When there is not enough water to circulate to these cells, the acid the cells produce will gradually and eventually erode the fine and detailed transcription patterns in the DNA repertoire stored in the cell nucleus. In time, the erosions can become permanent and disruptive, causing aberrant cells with the power to reproduce. These types of cells are more primitive and are locked into uncontrollable reproductive patterns.

For the benefit of those who want the scientific knowledge, in these cells the protein kinase C of normal cells gets converted to protein kinase M, which is an autonomous and unstoppable smaller enzyme that continues to stimulate cell reproduction without regard for boundary limitations. This is why cancer cells develop bulky masses and lumps that encroach on the adjacent tissues and interfere with the tissues' normal functions.

The DNA repair system is complex, and many different mechanisms are involved. One of these involves a small enzyme that has been discovered to cut and splice faulty DNA replications and correct the mistake. The enzyme is composed of lysine–tryptophan–lysine, discovered by Claude Helene, who published his findings in 1985. As has been explained, dehydration causes a drastic run on the tryptophan reserves of the body. Not only may the body be short of tryptophan, but the delivery of the amino acid to the microscopically dehydrated areas may also be a contributing factor and may affect the quality-control mechanisms for the DNA replication process.

Protein kinase enzymes are involved in manufacturing new proteins inside the cells. Proteases are a class of proteins that enzymatically break down already made proteins for their recycling process. This balancing process is going on in all the cells of the body all the time. If you exercise, you activate the enzymes for making new muscles. If you do not exercise, you activate the enzymes that break down already made muscles. In either case, water and the materials it normally transports play a major positive—or, if water and the materials are lacking, negative—role in this balancing process.

Dehydration has another impact on these enzymes. The protease activity and protein breakdown inside the cells become dominant in persistent dehydration. The cells produce fewer and fewer cell membrane receptors that would keep up communication with the physiological commands from different hormones in the body. The process is called receptor down-regulation. At a certain level of protease activity, the new class of protein-manufacturing enzyme known as protein kinase M, which is more befitting primitive cell functions, becomes produced. It is this enzyme that drives the cell into incessant reproduction. If you want more information on this topic, you can review my article "Receptor Down-Regulation" on www.watercure.com.

Unfortunately, medical experts in cancer research

have not understood the immune system suppression caused by persistent dehydration. It has not been realized that histamine can directly and indirectly suppress the immune system. When histamine is engaged in the drought-management programs of the body, it suppresses its own direct influence on the immune system, even at the bone marrow level. This is an essential process; the role of histamine in drought management could otherwise constantly flare up the immune system. As it happens, this safeguard may become ineffective and give rise to conditions known as lymphomas, myelomas, and leukemia.

The way excess histamine activity in persistent dehydration inhibits the immune system is simple. All the white cells in the body have histamine receptors. There are two major groups of white cells that are engaged in the immune system control mechanisms. They are known as helper cell and suppressor cell lymphocytes. There are twice as many suppressor cells in the bone marrow as there are helper cells. As their designation implies, the suppressor cells are there to inhibit any bone marrow manufacturing process. This is how inhibition of the role of the normal bone marrow activity within the immune system needs of the body is brought about, when the body is dehydrated.

Another major inhibitory effect of dehydration on the immune system is the role of vasopressin as a strong cortisone release factor. With increased cortisone activity, two things take place. First, more interleukin-1, a chemical produced by some white cells, is produced. Second, this chemical accentuates tissue breakdown for the release of raw materials from the protein reserves of the body. It also accentuates the action of cortisone in the inhibition of interleukin-2 and interferon production. These two elements are vital for efficient defensive functions of the immune system. They prime the cells that are on the forefront of the battle against infections, foreign agents, and aberrant cells that do not conform with the normal tissues of the body—such as cancer cells.

The function of interferon is crucial to the immune system. It causes a local release of hydrogen peroxide and ozone, which kill bacteria and cancer cells.

Scientists have for years tried to manufacture interferon for use in cancer treatment. What has been produced commercially has not worked as effectively as the natural form. Naturally, they did not realize that dehydration, and its other immune system impacts, should also be taken into consideration.

With this explanation on the direct impact of dehydration on tissue transformation and cancer production in the body, I am convinced that water is the best naturally preventive, and *curative*, cancer medication in the world. If you have any doubts about this, you can refer to my published scientific articles now posted on the Web site www.watercure.com.

When we wish to use water to help with cancers, we also need to provide the body with the right ingredients to correct the metabolic complications that have placed a depleting run on its raw material reserves. We also need to make sure that the body chemistry is directed toward a more *alkaline* state. Cancer cells are produced when the body becomes more and more acidic. Cancer cells are somewhat anaerobic; they do not like oxygen. In fact, oxygen is said to kill cancer cells. When water is available and brings with it all the defending agents and the needed ingredients, it also brings oxygen to the cancer cells. This is another reason why water is a good cancer medication.

For more information, take a look at my DVD or video *Health Miracles in Water and Salt.*

CHAPTER 12

THE WATER CURE: HOW MUCH WATER AND HOW OFTEN?

Let me give you the single most effective prescription for well-being, improved health, disease prevention, potentially reversible stages of degenerative diseases—and finally the best pain medicine in the world. It needs no doctor's prescription. It is freely available. It costs nothing. It has no dangerous side effects. It is the medication your body cries for when it is stressed. It is good old plain, natural *water*—ready cash for the industrial systems of the body.

Every twenty-four hours the body recycles the equivalent of forty thousand glasses of water to maintain its normal physiological functions. It does this every day of its life. Within this pattern of water metabolism and its recycling process, and depending on environmental conditions, the body becomes short of about six to ten glasses of water each day. This deficit has to be supplied to the body every day.

If you think you are different and your body does not need this amount of water, you are making a major mistake. The body uses up the equivalent of between six to eight glasses of its total body water for essential functions. It needs on average upwards of half its weight in ounces of water per day—a minimum of eight to ten glasses. Water should be taken in eight- or sixteen-ounce portions spaced throughout the day. In the same way you don't let your car run out of gas before you fill the tank, the body must not be allowed to become dehydrated before you drink water.

- Water should be drunk before meals. The optimum time is thirty minutes before eating. This prepares the digestive tract, particularly in people with gastritis, duodenitis, heartburn, peptic ulcer, colitis, or gas-producing indigestion.
- Water should be taken anytime you are thirsty— even during meals.
- Water should be taken two and a half hours after a meal to complete the process of digestion and correct the dehydration caused by food breakdown.
- Water should be taken first thing in the morning to correct dehydration produced during long sleep.
- Water should be taken before exercising to have it available for creating sweat.
- Water should be taken by people who are constipated and don't eat sufficient fruits and vegetables. Two to three glasses of water first thing in the morning act as a most effective laxative.

WATER OR FLUIDS?

Naturally, we wonder why we should drink water and not the pleasing and taste-enhancing beverages that are now the staples of our modern society. After all, they are made from water and do the job of quenching our thirst—or at least we feel they do. In fact, much of the problem of bad health is founded on this misconception. As far as the chemistry of the body is concerned, water and fluids are two different things. As it happens, popular manufactured beverages contain some chemicals that alter the body's chemistry at its central nervous system's control centers. Even milk is not the same as water. Milk is a food and must be treated as food.

The body needs water—nothing substitutes for water. Coffee, tea, soda, alcohol, and even milk and juices are not the same as water.

CAFFEINE IN BEVERAGES

- A cup of coffee contains about 80 milligrams of caffeine, and a cup of tea or one soda has about 50 milligrams.
- Chocolate also contains caffeine and theobromine, which acts like caffeine.
- Caffeine further dehydrates the body—you urinate more than the volume of water contained in the beverage.
- Caffeine blocks the production of melatonin in the brain. Dr. Kenneth Wright Jr. discovered the

melatonin-inhibiting effect of caffeine in 1994. This inhibitory effect of caffeine on melatonin production by the pineal gland of the brain seems to last six to nine hours. Melatonin regulates the functions of the body during sleep; it induces sleep. Thus, melatonin inhibition is one reason why coffee induces wakefulness.

- Caffeine intake on a regular basis by pregnant women can increase the risk of producing low-birth-weight infants. It can even cause spontaneous abortion or damage to the fetus.
- Caffeine inhibits the enzymes used in memory making, eventually causing loss of memory. It has been shown to inhibit the enzyme phosphodiesterase (phospho-di-esterase), which is involved in the process of learning and memory development.
- Caffeine can be toxic to brain cells. Some plants use caffeine as a defense against their predators. Caffeine toxicity in predators decreases their natural wit and ability for survival against their own predators. They forget how to camouflage themselves and become prey to their own predators. This is how the coffee plant gets rid of its pests.
- Seniors and children should not take caffeine. It can affect their normal brain functions, and their wit to survive may become less sharp.
- People taking five to six cups of coffee a day are twice as likely to suffer heart attacks.
- Caffeine can damage DNA and cause abnormal DNA by inhibiting the DNA-repair mechanism.
- Caffeine has been shown to cause genetic abnormalities in animals and plants.

- Caffeine attacks the brain cells' reserves of energy and lowers their threshold of control, so that the cells overspend from their energy pool. It indiscriminately turns on many energy-consuming functions to the point of causing exhaustion. When brain cells that have been influenced by caffeine confront a new situation that demands their full cooperation, they have a shortfall of energy. This creates a delay in brain response—hence exhaustion and irritability after excess caffeine consumption. Caffeine may cause attention deficit disorder in young people who consume too much soda.

- Water by itself generates hydroelectric energy. Caffeine in the same water stimulates the kidneys and causes more water to exit the body than is in the drink. This exhausts the brain cells' reserves of energy.

Caffeine-containing sodas with artificial sweeteners are more dangerous than those containing regular sugar. Artificial sweeteners are potent chemical agents that fool the brain cells by masking as sugar. Sweetness normally translates to the entry of energy into the body. The sweeteners, through the taste buds, program the brain to behave as if ample sugar for its consumption has reached the body and will imminently reach it through the circulation. Since there is strict control on the level of sugar in the blood, the brain calculates the outcome of the sweetness and instructs and programs the liver not to manufacture sugar from other raw materials, but to begin storing sugar. When the sugar that was promised through the taste buds is nowhere to be found, the brain and the liver prompt a hunger sensation to find food and make good on the promise of energy. The result is a state of anxiety about food. It has been shown that people who consume artificial sweeteners seek food, and eat more than normal, up to ninety minutes after the intake of the sweetener. This is part of the reason why more than 37 percent of the population is obese.

Caffeine-containing diet sodas, therefore, constitute a sort of double jeopardy to the body in that caffeine causes many complications, while artificial sweeteners have their own detrimental chemical effects. Decaffeinated diet sodas may be particularly harmful in diet programs, especially if the sweetener is aspartame. Aspartame has been implicated in the increased incidence of brain tumors and seizures.

ALCOHOL IN BEVERAGES

- Alcohol in beverages causes dehydration—the kidneys flush water out.
- Alcohol prevents the emergency water supply system to the brain. It inhibits the action of vasopressin and causes brain-cell dehydration. It is brain dehydration that signals as a hangover after you have taken a few drinks.
- Alcohol can be addictive and functionally depressive.
- Alcohol can cause impotence.
- Alcohol can cause liver damage.

- Alcohol can suppress the immune system.
- Alcohol consumption may increase the chances of developing cancers.
- Alcohol produces free radicals (acidlike substances) that normally attack and damage some sensitive tissues if allowed to circulate freely. Among other things, melatonin is used up to scavenge these free radicals. This results in low melatonin content in the body.
- Alcohol addiction may be caused in part by dehydration of cell membranes, particularly brain cells.
- Dehydration promotes the secretion of the natural endorphins in the body—the addictive factor.

Now that I have mentioned alcohol, let me also tell you that most alcoholics are actually searching for water. Water has a natural satiety impact through the hormones motilin, serotonin, and adrenaline, which culminates in the enhanced action of the body's endorphins. Alcoholics learn that alcohol, through its stressful dehydrating action on the brain, will also cause the release of endorphins. This is how they become addicted to alcohol. If alcoholics begin to increase their water intake, or reach for a glass of water in place of a beer or a shot of their favorite hard stuff, their cravings for alcohol will tend to decrease and they will be more likely to kick the habit with surprising ease.

The natural action of alcohol on the brain is an across-the-board inhibition of all its functions, including its pain-sensing centers. The inhibitory centers of the brain are depressed first. This is how some people get an emotional release in the presence of others from taking alcohol. If these people are by themselves, alcohol will probably put them to sleep. In short, *alcohol is a depressant.* Depressed people should not take it. Water, on the other hand, does not depress the brain, and it provides a more satisfying and enduring high, with lots of energy to perform whatever is desired.

JUICES AND MILK IN PLACE OF WATER

Replacing the water requirement of the body with juices or milk causes different problems. Too much orange juice increases histamine production and can cause asthma in children and adults. Even the natural sugar in juices will program the liver into fat-storing mode—a prescription for getting fat.

Milk should be considered a food. Infants who receive formulated milk other than mother's milk need it in a much more diluted form than is manufactured at present. Non-breast-fed babies should receive more water in their diet. It has been shown in some autopsies that infants who were not on mother's milk had developed heart arteries that showed signs of cholesterol. It is true that milk is a good watery source of calcium and proteins for health maintenance, yet milk should not be taken as a total replacement of the water that the body needs. It should be remembered that cow's milk is naturally designed for the calf that begins to walk within hours of its birth. To give undiluted milk to babies or children who are not moving much may be inviting trouble.

It is clear that the human body has many distinct ways of showing its general or local water needs, including its production of many localized complications such as asthma and allergies. Other drastic signs of the body's water needs are localized chronic pains such as heartburn, dyspepsia, rheumatoid joint pain, back pain, migraine headaches, leg pain when walking, colitis pain, and a most advanced sign, anginal pain. Complications such as hypertension, Alzheimer's disease, multiple sclerosis, muscular dystrophy, cholesterol blockage of the arteries (leading to heart attack and strokes), and diabetes may also be connected to dehydration. Ultimately, cancers, I believe, may also be a major health problem connected to persistent water shortage of the human body.

Chronic dehydration produces many symptoms, signs, and, eventually, the degenerative diseases. The physiological outcome of the sort of dehydration that produces any of the problems mentioned earlier in the book is almost the same. Different bodies manifest their early symptoms of drought differently, but in persistent dehydration that has been camouflaged by prescription medications, one by one the other symptoms and signs will kick in, and eventually the person will suffer from multiple "diseases."

We in medicine have labeled these conditions as outright "diseases" or have grouped them as different "syndromes." In recent years, we have grouped some of the syndromes—with some typical blood tests—and called them autoimmune diseases, such as lupus, multiple sclerosis, muscular dystrophy, insulin-independent diabetes, and so on.

Medical research has until now been conducted on the assumption that many conditions—which I consider to be states of dehydration or its complications—are diseases of unknown etiology. From the presently held perspectives of human health problems, we are not allowed to use the word *cure*. We can at best "treat" a problem and hope it goes "into remission."

From my perspective, most painful degenerative diseases are states of local or regional drought—with varying patterns. It naturally follows that, once the drought is corrected, the problem will be cured if the dehydration damage is not extensive. I also believe that to evaluate deficiency disorders—water deficiency being one of them—we do not need to observe the same research protocols that are applied to the research of chemical products. Identifying the shortage and correcting the deficiency is all we have to do.

It is now clear that the treatment for all dehydration-produced conditions is the same—a single treatment protocol for umpteen number of conditions. Isn't that great? One program solves so many problems and avoids costly and unnecessary interferences with the body.

The first step in this treatment program involves a clear and determined upward adjustment of daily water intake. Persistent dehydration also causes a disproportionate loss of certain elements that should be adequately available in the stored reserves in the body. Naturally, the ideal treatment protocol will also involve an appropriate correction of the associated metabolic disturbance. In short, treatment of dehydration-produced diseases also involves correction of the secondary deficiencies that water deficiency imposes on some tissues of the body. This multiple-deficiency phenomenon, caused by dehydration, is at the root of many degenerative diseases.

A change of lifestyle becomes vital for the correction of any dehydration-produced disorder. The backbone of The Water Cure program is, simply, sufficient water and salt intake; regular exercise; a balanced, mineral-rich diet that includes lots of fruits and vegetables and the essential fats needed to create cell membranes, hormones, and nerve insulation; exclusion of caffeine and alcohol; and meditation to solve and detoxify stressful thoughts. Exclusion of artificial sweeteners from the diet is an absolute must for better health.

It should also be remembered that the sort of dehydration that manifests itself as asthma leaves other scars within the interior parts of the human body. This is why asthma in childhood is such a devastating condition that leaves its mark on children and may expose them to many different health problems in later life. My understanding of the serious damaging effects of dehydration during childhood is the reason I have been concentrating much of my efforts on the eradication of asthma among children.

The first nutrient the body needs is water. *Water is a nutrient. It generates energy.* Water dissolves all the minerals, proteins, starch, and other water-soluble components and, as blood, carries them around the body for distribution. Think of blood as seawater that has a few species of fish in it—red cells, white cells, platelets, proteins, and enzymes that swim to a destination. The blood serum has almost the same mineral consistency and proportions as seawater.

The human body is in constant need of water. It loses water through the lungs when we breathe out. It loses water in perspiration, in urine production, and in daily bowel movements. A good gauge for the water needs of the body is the color of urine. A well-hydrated person produces colorless urine—not counting the color of vitamins or color additives in food. A comparatively dehydrated person produces yellow urine. A truly dehydrated person produces urine that is orange in color. An exception is those who are on diuretics and flush water out of their already dehydrated bodies and yet produce colorless urine.

The body needs no less than two quarts of water and a half teaspoon of salt every day to compensate for its natural losses in urine, respiration, and perspiration. Less than this amount will place a burden on the kidneys. They will have to work harder to concentrate the urine and excrete as much chemical toxic waste in as little water as possible. This process is highly taxing to the kidney cells. A rough rule of thumb for those who are heavyset is to drink a half ounce of water for every pound of body weight. A two-hundred-pound person will need to take one hundred ounces of water. Water should be taken anytime you are thirsty, even in the middle of a meal. Water intake in the middle of a meal does not drastically affect the process of digestion, but dehydration during food intake does. You should also take at least two glasses of water first thing in the morning to correct for water loss during eight hours of sleep.

CHAPTER 13

MINERALS ARE VITAL

Certain minerals need to pass through the acidic environment of the stomach before they can be absorbed through the mucosa of the intestine. They are *zinc, magnesium, manganese, selenium, iron, copper, chromium,* and *molybdenum.* The list is in the order, in my view, of each element's importance to the human body. The mineral elements that the body needs in largest quantities are sodium, potassium, calcium, and magnesium.

Sodium will enforce the osmotic needs and balance of the fluid environment outside and around the cells of the body, vitally important to brain function. If someone overhydrates and forces salt out of the body without replacing it, the brain cells will gradually swell up; the person could suffer brain damage and die. This happens from time to time if people exercise regularly, sweat profusely and lose salt, and then keep on drinking only water without replacing the lost salt. As I have said repeatedly, salt is not bad for you. It does not raise the blood pressure. It is the insufficiency of other minerals that normally hold on to and keep water inside the cells that causes a rise in blood pressure. Given in conjunction with other minerals, salt will actually lower blood pressure to normal levels.

Potassium, calcium, magnesium, and zinc are the main minerals that regulate the water levels inside the cells. These elements are needed to keep the interior of the cells in the body in osmotic balance and in good working order. These are the elements that work with sodium to keep blood pressure in its normal range.

All one-a-day vitamin supplements are now composed in such a way that the daily requirements of the essential minerals—other than sodium, calcium, and potassium—are provided. The rest of the vital minerals are fully available in the variety of foods we eat. Vitamin and mineral supplements are thus recommended for insurance in case your daily diet is not high quality and contains insufficient fruits and vegetables.

The toxic mineral elements are mercury, lead, aluminum, arsenic, cadmium, and, in large quantities, iron. These minerals should be avoided—they are absorbed better by the body if the stomach is less acidic than normal.

As we grow older, some of us manufacture less and less acid in our stomachs. The condition is called achlorhydria. People with achlorhydria can become deficient of vital minerals in their bodies. They also have difficulty in digesting meat.

In older cultures, eating pickles with food was a precautionary measure to prevent this problem. The use of vinegar in salads eaten with meals has the same effect, if the salad dressing is sour in taste. If the meal contains a lot of meat, the stomach normally secretes plenty of acid to break down the meat into small digestible particles. These smaller particles are then further reduced to the size of their amino acid components in the intestines and get absorbed. People who have difficulty digesting food should get into the habit of taking some lemon or pickles with their food.

A good pickle for this purpose would be finely chopped cauliflower, green tomatoes, carrots, celery, onion, mushrooms, eggplant, and cabbage, with salt and pepper. The ingredients should be put in a jar, covered with a good vinegar, and left for a few days to season. When eaten, the small vinegar-soaked particles will mix with the food in the stomach and acidify their immediate vicinity for the enzymes to become activated for digestion. Middle Eastern food markets have these kinds of pickled foods available for ready use.

SALT: THE ETERNAL MEDICATION

Salt is a vital substance for the survival of all living creatures, particularly humans, and especially people with asthma, allergies, and autoimmune disease.

Salt is a "medication" that has been used by healers throughout the ages. In certain cultures, it is worth its weight in gold and is, in fact, exchanged weight for weight for gold. In desert countries, people know that salt intake is their insurance for survival. To these people, salt mines are synonymous with gold mines.

After many years of salt being badmouthed by ignorant health professionals and their media parrots, the importance of salt as a dietary supplement is once again being acknowledged and recognized. I was one of the early voices bringing about this change.

Water, salt, and potassium together regulate the water content of the body. Water regulates the water content of the interior of the cell by working its way into all the cells it reaches. It has to get there to cleanse and extract the toxic waste of cell metabolism. Once water gets into the cells, the potassium content of the cells holds on to it and keeps it there—to the extent that potassium is available inside the cells. Even in the plant kingdom, it is potassium in the fruit that gives it firmness by holding water in the interior of the fruit. Our daily food contains ample potassium from its natural sources of fruits and vegetables, but not salt from its natural source. That is why we need to add salt to our daily diet. Note: Do not take too much potassium as a dietary supplement. It could cause trouble.

Salt forces some water to keep it company outside the cells (osmotic retention of water by salt). It balances the amount of water that is held outside the cells.

Basically, there are two oceans of water in the body: One is held inside the cells of the body, and the other is held outside. Good health depends on a most delicate balance between the volumes of these two oceans. This balance is achieved by the regular intake of water, potassium-rich fruits and vegetables that also contain the vitamins needed by the body, and salt. Unrefined sea salt, which contains some of the other minerals that the body needs, is preferable. Sea salt may not contain enough iodine to keep the thyroid gland working normally, and it may enlarge into a goiter. Regular intake of a multivitamin that contains iodine is essential. Another source of iodine is dried kelp capsules, which are available from vitamin shops.

When water is not available to get into the cells freely, it is filtered from the outside salty ocean and injected into cells that are being overworked despite their water shortage. This secondary and emergency means of supplying important cells with injected water is the reason, in severe dehydration, that we retain salt and develop edema—to have more water available to draw from for filtration and injection into the cells.

The design of our bodies is such that the extent of the ocean of water outside the cells is expanded to have extra water in reserve for filtration and emergency injection into vital cells. To achieve this, the brain commands an increase in salt and water retention by the kidneys. This directive of the brain is the reason we get edema when we don't drink enough water.

When water shortage in the body reaches a more critical level, and delivery of water by its injection into the cells becomes the main route of supply to more and more cells, an associated rise in injection pressure becomes necessary. The significant rise in pressure needed to inject water into the cells becomes measurable and is labeled "hypertension," or high blood pressure.

Initially, the process of water filtration and its delivery into the cells is more efficient at night when the body is horizontal. In this position, the collected water, which settles mostly in the legs during the day, does not have to fight the force of gravity to get into the blood circulation. If reliance on this process of emergency hydration of some cells continues for long, the lungs begin to get waterlogged at night, and breathing becomes difficult. The person needs more pillows to sit upright to sleep. This condition is called cardiac asthma, and it is the consequence of dehydration. However, in this condition you must not overload the system by drinking too much water at the beginning. Increases in water intake must be slow and spaced out—until urine production begins to increase at the same rate that you drink water.

When we drink enough water to pass clear urine, we also pass out a lot of the salt that was held back. This is how we can get rid of edema fluid from the body. Not by diuretics, but by more water! Water is the best natural diuretic that exists.

In a person who has extensive edema and whose heart sometimes beats irregularly or rapidly with little effort, the increase in water intake should be gradual and spaced out, but water should not be withheld from the body. Salt intake should be limited for two or three days because the body is still in an overdrive mode to retain it. Once the edema has cleared, salt should again be added to the diet. If there are irregular heartbeats, or the pulse is fast and furious but there is no edema, increased water, salt, and other minerals such as magnesium, calcium, and some potassium will alleviate the problem.

SALT: SOME OF ITS HIDDEN MIRACLES

Salt has many other important functions than just regulating the water content of the body.

- Salt is a strong natural antihistamine. It can be used to relieve asthma: Put it on the tongue after drinking a glass or two of water. It is as effective as an inhaler, without the toxicity. You should drink one or two glasses of water before putting salt on the tongue. *This type of salt use is only for emergencies.* Normally you should add it to food or to water before drinking it.
- Salt is a strong antistress element for the body.
- Salt is vital for extracting excess acidity from inside the cells, particularly the brain cells. If you don't want Alzheimer's disease, don't go salt-free and don't let them put you on diuretic medications for long!
- Salt is vital for the kidneys to clear excess acidity and pass the acidity into the urine. Without sufficient salt in the body, the body will become more and more acidic.
- Salt is essential in the treatment of emotional and affective disorders. Lithium is a salt substitute that is used in the treatment of depression.
- Salt is essential for preserving the serotonin and melatonin levels in the brain. When water and salt perform their natural antioxidant duties and clear the toxic waste from the body, essential amino acids, such as tryptophan and tyrosine, will not be sacrificed as chemical antioxidants. In a well-

hydrated body, tryptophan is spared and gets into the brain tissue, where it is used to manufacture serotonin, melatonin, and tryptamine—essential antidepressant neurotransmitters.

- Salt, in my opinion, is vital for the prevention and treatment of cancer. Cancer cells are killed by oxygen; they are anaerobic organisms. They must live in a low-oxygen environment. When the body is well hydrated and salt expands the volume of blood circulation to reach all parts of the body, the oxygen and the active and motivated immune cells in the blood reach the cancerous tissue and destroy it. As I have explained, dehydration— shortage of water and salt—suppresses the immune system and the activity of its disease-fighting cells in the body.

- Salt is vital for maintaining muscle tone and strength. Lack of bladder control and involuntary leakage of urine could be a consequence of low salt intake. The following letter from Dottlee Reid, in her sixties, speaks volumes. It reveals how salt intake helped her get over a knee problem as well as constant involuntaiy leakage of urine. I have chosen to print this letter here to share with millions of senior citizens in America—who might be on diuretics—the good news that adequate salt intake can possibly save them from the embarrassment of having to constantly wear pads.

Dear Doctor Batmanghelidj:

June 25, 1999, I had to go home from work because the pain in my knee became unbearable. (This was an old wound, years ago caused by a chiropractor, that had been bruised again.) I was staying in bed a lot as it was too painful to try to walk.

I got your book and tapes (Your Body's Many Cries for Water). By July 3, 1999, I decided to try to walk around the block. I made it and July 4, 1999, I walked six blocks to church. On July 5, 1999, I rode in the car for seven hours, only stopping twice to use the rest room. I have a very weak bladder and had even taken spare clothing as I was sure they would be needed. I arrived with not a drop of anything on my clothing, and for the first time in my life was not tired and I even took a walk before I went to bed.

I was very thin and was limited on what I could eat. Suddenly I find I am eating things I have not been able to eat in years—peaches, cantaloupe, watermelon, tomatoes, pineapple, and even sweets—and I was enjoying them with no side effects.

I had not been drinking anything but water for years, but I had talked myself off salt. A bad mistake! My muscles were really screaming as well as many parts of my body. I still have problems to be worked out, but I'm learning how to listen to my own body and I hope to see the day I won't have any more problems with gas, digestion, circulation, and allergies. I can truthfully say most days I do feel better than I have in many years, and I can never thank you enough for your help.

- Salt can be very effective in stabilizing irregular heartbeats and, contrary to the misconception that it causes high blood pressure, is actually essential for the regulation of blood pressure—in conjunction with water and the minerals I have mentioned. Naturally, the proportions are critical. A low-salt diet with high water intake will, in some people, actually cause the blood pressure to rise. The logic is simple. If you drink water and do not take salt, the water will not stay in the blood circulation adequately to completely fill all the blood vessels. In some, this will cause fainting; in others, it will cause tightening of the arteries to the point of registering a rise in blood pressure. One or two glasses of water and some salt—a little of it on the tongue—will quickly and efficiently quiet a racing and "thumping" heart and, in the long run, will reduce the blood pressure. Talk with your doctor about the right balance of water and salt for your diet.
- Salt is vital for sleep regulation. It is a natural hypnotic. If you drink a full glass of water, then put a few grains of salt on your tongue and let it stay there, you will fall into a natural, deep sleep. Don't use salt on your tongue unless you also drink water. Repeated use of salt by itself might cause nosebleeds. Routine intake of water and the *addition of some salt to the diet* will regulate the sleep pattern.
- Salt is a vitally needed element for diabetics. It helps balance the sugar levels in the blood and reduces the need for insulin in those who have to inject it to regulate their blood sugar levels. Water and salt can reduce the extent of secondary damage

to the eyes and the blood vessels associated with diabetes.

- Salt is vital for the generation of hydroelectric energy in all of the cells in the body. It is used for local power generation at the sites of energy need by the cells.
- Salt is vital to the communication and information processing of nerve cells the entire time that the brain cells work—from the moment of conception to death.
- Salt is vital for the absorption of food particles through the intestinal tract.
- Salt is vital for clearing the lungs of mucus plugs and sticky phlegm, particularly in asthma, emphysema, and cystic fibrosis sufferers.
- Salt on the tongue can help stop persistent dry coughs.
- Salt is vital for clearing up catarrh and sinus congestion.
- Salt can help in the prevention of gout and gouty arthritis.
- Salt is essential for preventing muscle cramps.
- Salt is vital in preventing excess saliva production to the point that it flows out of the mouth during sleep. Needing to constantly mop up excess saliva indicates a salt shortage.
- Osteoporosis may be the result of a salt and water shortage in the body.
- Salt is absolutely vital to making the structure of bones firm.
- Salt can help you maintain self-confidence and a positive self-image—a serotonin- and melatonin-controlled personality output.

- Salt can help maintain libido.
- Salt may help reduce a double chin. When the body is short of salt, it means the body really is short of water. The salivary glands sense the salt shortage and are obliged to produce more saliva to lubricate the act of chewing and swallowing and also to supply the stomach with the water that it needs for breaking down foods. Circulation to the salivary glands increases, and the blood vessels become "leaky" in order to supply the glands with more water to manufacture saliva. This leakiness spills to areas beyond the glands themselves, causing increased bulk under the skin of the chin and the cheeks and into the neck.
- Salt may help prevent varicose veins and spider veins on the legs and thighs.
- Sea salt contains about eighty mineral elements that the body needs. Some of these elements are needed in trace amounts. Unrefined sea salt is a better choice than other types of salt on the market. Ordinary table salt that is bought in the supermarkets has been stripped of its companion elements and might contain additive elements such as aluminum silicate to keep it powdery and porous. Aluminum is a very toxic element in our nervous system. It has been implicated as one of the primary causes of Alzheimer's disease. Sea salt is not rich in iodine, which needs to be taken as a supplement.

As much as salt is good for the body in asthma, excess potassium is bad for it. Too much orange juice, too many bananas, or any sports drink containing too much potassium might help precipitate an asthma attack, particularly if too much of the drink or too many bananas are taken before exercising. It can cause an exercise-induced asthma attack. To prevent such attacks, some salt intake before exercise will increase the lungs' capacity for air exchange. It will also decrease excess sweating.

It is a good policy to add some salt to orange juice to balance the actions of sodium and potassium in maintaining the required volume of water inside and outside the cells. In some cultures, salt is added to melon and other fruits to accentuate their sweetness. In effect, these fruits contain mostly potassium. By adding salt to them before eating, a balance between the intake of sodium and potassium results. The same should be done to other juices.

I received a call one day from one of my readers to tell me how he had unwittingly hurt his son. Knowing that orange juice was full of vitamin C, he forced his son to drink several glasses of it every day. The boy developed breathing problems and had a number of asthma attacks until he reached college and moved out of the sphere of influence of his father. His asthma then cleared and his breathing became normal. The father told me he had to call his son and apologize for having given him such a hard time when he was younger. The more the son had rebelled against orange juice, the more the father had insisted he should take it, convinced a large amount was good for him.

As a rough rule of thumb, you need about 3 to 4 grams of salt a day for every ten glasses of water you drink. Three grams is about a half teaspoon. An easier calculation is a quarter teaspoon of salt per quart of water (I know someone who takes more than a tea-spoon of salt every day to control his asthma). You should take salt throughout the day. If you exercise and sweat, you need more salt. In hot climates, when you lose water from the surface of the skin without realizing it, you need to take even more salt. In these climates, salt can make the difference between survival and better health and heat exhaustion and death.

Warning! At the same time, you must not overdo salt. You must observe the ratio of salt and water needs of the body. Always make sure you drink enough water to wash the excess salt out of the body. If your weight suddenly goes up in one day when you have not con-sumed too much food, you have taken too much salt. Hold back on salt intake for one day and drink plenty of water to increase your urine output and get rid of your swelling. Consult your doctor to determine the correct balance of salt and water for your diet.

If you begin to drink water according to my pro-tocol, you might also benefit from taking a one-a-day vitamin tablet daily, particularly if you do not exercise or eat hearty portions of vegetables and fruits. Meat and fish proteins are good sources of selenium and zinc. If you are under stress, and until it is over, you might consider adding some vitamin B_6 and zinc to your diet in addition to what is available in the vitamin tablets.

If you suffer from cold sores (herpes simplex virus on the lips and even in the eyes) or genital herpes, make sure you add zinc and vitamin B_6 to your diet. Your viral sores might very well be the result of zinc deficiency and its associated complications.

CHAPTER 14

OTHER ESSENTIALS FOR HEALTH AND HEALING

While water, salt, and minerals are vital for optimal health, the nutrients we receive from the foods we eat are also important, as is the need to stay fit through regular exercise. In this chapter, I will give a brief overview of the other essentials—proteins, fats, fruits, vegetables, sunlight, and exercise—needed for optimal health and healing.

PROTEINS

Many experts are of the opinion that the body needs a minimum of between 1.1 and 1.4 grams of good-quality protein for every kilogram—2.2 pounds—of body weight per day. A 200-pound (90 kg) person thus needs about 4.5 ounces—120 grams—of protein a day to maintain muscle mass. At this level of protein intake, the body will retain its normal composition of protein reserves and will not break into them and deplete some of the amino acid reserves.

Children need a basic minimum of about 1 gram of protein for every pound of body weight.

You must bear in mind that the protein portion of high-protein foods varies from source to source. For example: An egg weighs about 50 grams and has only 6 grams of pure protein; meat contains 7 grams of pure protein in every ounce; hard cheeses contain about 7 grams of pure protein per ounce; soft cheeses contain about 3 grams of pure protein per ounce; tofu contains about 5 grams of pure protein per ounce. One ounce is 28.3 grams. In other words, not all the weight of the protein foods is pure protein.

In advanced societies that place high demands for increased productivity on their labor force and have no food shortages, the recommended regular intake of protein seems to be much higher. The more physically active you are, the more protein-containing food your body needs. The extra protein is needed for tissue repairs and the manufacture of enzymes and neurotransmitters. High-protein diets are now fashionable in weight-loss programs.

STRESS AND AMINO ACIDS

It is my published opinion that continued *submissive endurance of stress* depletes the body of certain absolutely essential amino acids—tryptophan, tyrosine, cysteine, and methionine in particular. These amino acids must be present in correct proportions for the body's main functions to take place in a coordinated manner. This is a part of what I mean by the regulation of the body as an integrated system. Let us see some aspects of what these amino acids mean to the body. Then we may understand the impact of stress and be alert to its main signals in the body.

Before we get into the discussion of the individual amino acids, let me give you some basic information. There are twenty different amino acids from which proteins are made up. By selectively mixing the amino acids, some more than others, different proteins are manufactured. The manufactured proteins have different shapes and sizes, and are three-dimensional structures that twist and rotate all the time. During these twists and rotations they present different facets that become attractive to their chemically predetermined partners, and a desired response is generated when they unite or have an effect on each other. It is from the sum total of these desired responses that life and actions of all living matter come into being.

The food that we eat provides not only some of the energy needed to function, but also some of the basic amino acids as raw materials for protein production. In more dilute solutions, the proteins and enzymes of the body develop a greater movement and rotational freedom and become more efficient in finding and coupling with their chemical partners. Thus, dehydration can cause a slowing of these natural movements and could be responsible for the slowing of body reactions and loss of certain sensations as we grow older and become more dehydrated.

The human body can manufacture twelve of the twenty amino acids from other raw materials, but needs to import into the system eight of them to be able to manufacture the complete range of its protein and neurotransmitter needs. These "imports" are called essential amino acids. Without them, and in an exact sufficiency at that, the body will not function. I use the words *exact sufficiency* to indicate that more is not better. Just because these amino acids are essential does not mean we should load the body with them. This attitude is dangerous. The rate of assimilation of one amino acid depends on the presence of the others in proportionate amounts. The excess presence of one can have a disruptive effect and alter the metabolism rate of the others. So beware of buying amino acids that are manufactured and sold by the bottle.

The essential amino acids are *isoleucine, leucine, lysine, methionine, phenylalanine, threonine, tryptophan,* and *valine*. Since tyrosine is manufactured from phenylalanine and cysteine is manufactured from methionine, *tyrosine* and *cysteine* should also be considered essential amino acids. There are limits to the rate of manufacture of *arginine* and *histidine* in the young and the old, so, in essence, these amino acids are also to be considered essential. In effect, there are twelve essential amino acids that the body needs to import at various stages of its development if its normal functions are to be guaranteed. I will deal with only a few of them to explain some aspects of the metabolism disturbance in chronic dehydration and stress.

Tryptophan is an essential amino acid that is highly sensitive to heat. It spins at a much faster rate when the temperature of the body rises even a few degrees. It seems to respond to the heat of activation produced by water. It performs certain functions more efficiently when there is more water in the body, particularly when water is essential to activate the hydroelectric pump units in the cell membrane and generate energy and heat. The mechanism involved in the passage of tryptophan through the wall of the blood vessels of the brain is complicated. However, the consistency of blood, on the dilute side, enormously helps the passage of tryptophan into the brain and the centers of its activity. Tryptophan gives rise to the neurotransmitter agent serotonin, along with its deputies tryptamine and melatonin.

Tryptophan also has a natural role in recognizing and repairing damaged, unnatural, and inexact DNA structures. DNA is the material at the center of re-creation of life from one living matter into another. The secrets of re-creation are held in the DNA content of the body. Its correct representation is essential to give rise to the next generation, be it the daughter cell in an organ or the next-generation offspring. It is my view that cancer cells are daughter cells that have transformed into faulty new cells because the DNA-repair system has become inadequate due to a breakdown in the tryptophan-regulatory process. Dr. Jawed Iqbal, a world-recognized cancer researcher who lives in England, has studied the scientific explanations for the above statement. After much scrutiny, he has accepted the validity of the concept and has written a number of articles that can be viewed in the section on science on the Web site www.watercure.com.

It has now been recognized that tryptophan forms a tripod team with two units of lysine, another amino acid, and forms an enzyme that acts as the quality controller on the DNA assembly line. It seems that tryptophan projection of the enzyme is responsible for cutting and repairing any damaged site in the DNA assembly.

As far as the brain is concerned, as soon as tryptophan reaches the brain side of the circulation it becomes converted into the various neurotransmitters. Research seems to indicate that almost all of the problems of the human body become established when the rate of entry of tryptophan to the brain centers that use the neurotransmitter derivatives of tryptophan is negatively affected.

My research indicates a direct relationship between the level of water in the body and the rate of tryptophan transfer across the blood–brain barrier. In dehydration, less tryptophan gets across. The level of tryptophan entry into the brain determines the intensity of the pain sensation. When there is less tryptophan, the pain sensation registers more intensely. With increased tryptophan getting into the brain, the pain sensation decreases until it disappears. The relationship of the thirst signal in the body to the feeling of pain associated with thirst seems to indicate a decrease in tryptophan entry into the brain. In this way the pain associated with a certain level of dehydration, beyond the threshold of rationing the available water and adaptation to chronic dehydration, explains the way pain registers when there is dehydration.

In stress dehydration, more tryptophan in its free form is released from the reserves of the body. The liver has a metering system for free tryptophan. When it reaches a certain level, the liver begins to recycle and destroy it and finally discard its by-products. This is a very drastic way of getting rid of an essential amino acid. It has to be done, however, because in its free form tryptophan is used in other capacities, such as in a substitute cleaning process when water is not available to wash away the toxic waste.

When used in this way, stress-initiated breakdown of tryptophan can deplete the reserves of this most essential amino acid in the body. It is to prevent this event that, in any form of stress, you should immediately begin to drink copious amounts of water. This is why dehydration causes stress—and stress precipitates so many disease conditions in the body. Tryptophan is involved in the formation of the color of the iris of the eye. It acts as filter to intense light and ultraviolet rays that might damage the retina.

Another important effect of tryptophan on proper metabolism is in muscle movement. Large muscles of the body demonstrate an avid metabolism for the branched chain amino acids *valine*, *leucine*, and *isoleucine*, three of the twenty amino acids in the body. During exercise and movement of the large muscle mass, these three amino acids are used up for their energy content. They also compete with tryptophan for passage across the blood–brain barrier and entry to the brain. Unless tryptophan enters into the brain tissue, a state of calm and peace will not prevail. The importance of exercise—walking at least one hour a day—cannot be stressed enough. *It is as a result of burning these competitors of tryptophan by the muscle tissue that a well-regulated physiology in the body can be established.*

Tyrosine is another most important and responsible amino acid in the human body. It is the base material for the manufacture of adrenaline and noradrenaline—the neurotransmitters that coordinate the action-oriented functions of the body. Tyrosine is also essential for the manufacture of the neurotransmitter dopamine, of the thyroid hormones, and of the skin pigment called melanin, the suntan pigment. This amino acid is also critical for the composition of certain essential proteins, including the insulin receptor.

In stress, the enzyme that breaks up tyrosine becomes excessively activated. If the enzyme is allowed to continue its run on the body's reserve of tyrosine beyond the rate of its manufacture, certain essential functions become severely affected. Tyrosine and tryptophan seem to be excessively destroyed when there is dehydration/stress in the body.

Sources of Good Proteins

Good-quality proteins can be found in eggs, milk, and legumes. Legumes such as lentils, mung beans, broad beans, and soy beans are 24 percent high-quality proteins. Vegetables also contain good-quality protein (spinach is about 13 percent protein), as do fresh turkey, chicken, veal, beef, pork, and fish. I use the word *fresh* because animal meat contains different enzymes that quickly destroy some of the essential amino acids within its proteins. Prolonged exposure to oxygen also destroys some of the essential amino acids in meat proteins. It makes the good fats in meat rancid and useless to the body.

Do not take individual amino acids as supplements instead of a balanced protein diet. At a certain concentration, some have adverse effects on the mineral and vitamin balance of the body. Amino acids in the body function more efficiently when they are proportionately represented.

Eggs are a wholesome food. An average egg weighs 50 grams and has an energy value of eighty calories. The white of an egg weighs about 33 grams and the yolk about 17 grams. Eggs contain about 6 grams of top-quality proteins, no carbohydrates, and no fiber. The protein content of eggs is composed of a balanced range of amino acids. Eggs are rich in vitamins such as biotin and minerals such as manganese, selenium, phosphorus, and copper. The yolk is a rich source of sulfur, a natural antioxidant that is now recognized as vital for health and well-being.

About 10 percent of an egg is its lipid or fat content. The lipid composition of the egg yolk is unique. It is rich in both lecithin, which is the precursor of the neurotransmitter acetylcholine, and docosahexaenoic acid (DHA). DHA is an essential fat for maintaining brain function. It is needed for the constant repair of brain-cell membranes and their cell-to-cell contact points—synaptosomes. The nerve structure of the eyes uses much DHA for interpreting colors and for quality and sharpness of vision. Apart from being found in eggs, DHA is also found in cold-water fish and algae.

It is being increasingly understood that the level of

cholesterol in the circulation is not affected by a high-egg diet. It is a medically published fact that an elderly man has for many years eaten about twenty-four eggs a week without any clinically significant rise in his cholesterol level.

The next time you come across a person who talks about "bad cholesterol" being the cause of heart disease, ask: "Is it not true that we measure the cholesterol levels in the body in the blood that is drawn from a vein?" If it is true that the cholesterol level is the cause of plaques and obstruction of the blood vessels, when a slower rate of blood flow would encourage further cholesterol deposits, then we should also see more blockage of the veins of the body. Since there is not a single scientific report of cholesterol deposits causing blockage of the veins, the assumption that cholesterol is "bad" and is the cause of heart disease is erroneous and unscientific.

Let me again explain why we get cholesterol deposits in the arteries of the heart or the brain or even on the inner wall of the major arteries of the body. Remember, the term *dehydration* really refers to concentrated, acidic blood. Acidic blood that is also concentrated pulls water out of the cells lining the arterial wall. At the same time, the fast rush of blood against the delicate cells lining the inner wall of the arteries, weakened by loss of their water and damaged by constant toxicity of concentrated blood, produces microscopic abrasions.

Another of the many functions of cholesterol is its use as a sort of waterproof dressing to cover the damaged sites within the arterial membranes until they are repaired. Cholesterol acts as a sort of waterproof covering—a "grease gauze"—that protects the inner wall of the artery from rupturing and peeling off. When you look at cholesterol through this perspective, you will realize what a blessing it really is. This particular action of cholesterol is actually designed to save the lives of people whose bodies get seriously damaged as a result of persistent dehydration.

In my opinion, all the statistics about the level of cholesterol in the blood and the number of people who die of heart disease reflect the extent of the killer dehydration that has also caused the level of blood cholesterol to rise.

Another most important role of cholesterol in the body will be discussed later in this chapter. Based on this new understanding of cholesterol, I have no hesitation in recommending eggs as a very good source of the essential dietary needs of the human body.

Milk Products

For people who can digest milk products, natural, unsweetened yogurt is a good source of high-quality protein. It also contains lots of vitamins and good bacteria. The good bacteria in yogurt keep the intestinal tract healthy and help prevent the growth of toxic bacteria and toxic yeasts such as candida. Of course, people who are allergic to dairy products should not take yogurt.

Cheeses are also a good source of protein. Freshly prepared cheeses are easier to digest and, in my opinion, are more wholesome than aged cheeses. Some people cannot digest cow's milk easily. Soy milk is a very good substitute. If you do not like the taste of soy milk, mix it with carrot juice and enjoy the advantage of additional vitamins and nutrients. The combination is healthy and tasty.

ESSENTIAL FATS

Fat is an essential dietary requirement of the body. Some vital fatty acids that make up certain fats and oils are used as primary materials in the manufacture of cell membranes. They are also primary ingredients from which many of the hormones of the body are manufactured. The manufacture of sex hormones depends on the presence of some essential fats in the body, including the much-maligned cholesterol. Nerve cells need the "good" fats to remanufacture their constantly used-up nerve endings.

The essential fat components are omega-6—a polyunsaturated fatty acid known as linoleic acid— and omega-3, which is a superunsaturated fatty acid known as alpha-linolenic acid. These fatty acids are in the form of oils. Our bodies cannot manufacture these essential fatty acids and have to import them in the form of oils in food.

The average body needs, absolutely, between 6 and 9 grams of linoleic acid a day. It also needs around 2 to 9 grams of alpha-linolenic acid (omega-3), the most essential of the fatty acids. These fatty acids are needed particularly by the brain cells and their long nerves to manufacture insulated membranes that need to be impermeable and prevent interference to the rate and flow of neurotransmission. The nerve endings in the retina that are involved in object recognition and clarity of sight have a high turnover of these essential fatty acids, particularly DHA. DHA is made from omega-3 fatty acid and is vital for brain-cell composition. People with neurological disorders have been shown to be short of DHA.

As mentioned, eggs, cold-water fish, and algae are good sources of DHA. Another excellent source of the omega-3 and omega-6 fatty acids, in an ideal ratio of 3:1, is flaxseed oil (also known as linseed oil) that is cold-pressed and bottled in dark containers that keep out light. A similar oil is grapeseed oil. Light destroys these essential oils, which is why they are also packed in dark capsules. Sesame oil has the desirable property of being highly unsaturated. It is the eating oil of choice in many ancient cultures. Canola oil is also a good source of some essential fatty acids. The reason oils are better than solid fats is because at normal body temperature they remain as oils and do not turn into sticky lard.

For detailed information on the essential fatty acids and their best sources, refer to the book *Fats That Heal, Fats That Kill*, by Dr. Udo Erasmus. Another good and readable book on this topic is *Smart Fats*, by Dr. Michael A. Schmidt. I also recommend a book on vitamins and minerals that I found easy reading with lots of useful information. It is *The Complete Illustrated Guide to Vitamins and Minerals* by Denise Mortimer.

Butter is a rich source of fat-soluble vitamins, such

as vitamin K, vitamin A, vitamin E, lecithin, folic acid, and more. Butter is also a rich source of calcium and phosphorous. The body needs some fat in its daily diet. You cannot go fat-free and survive for long. The body is not able to manufacture certain fat components that are needed to make its insulating membranes. If you don't give the body what it needs, it will try to make the required element from the carbohydrate content in its daily diet. However, since the body is unable to complete the process of making essential fats, it proceeds to store the unfinished product. This is how some people grow disproportionately fat. If you want to lose weight, your diet must contain some fat. Each gram of fat provides the body with nine calories of energy. Recent studies have confirmed the importance of adequate fat in diets designed for weight loss.

FRUITS, VEGETABLES, AND SUNLIGHT

The body also needs fruits and green vegetables daily. They are ideal sources of the natural vitamins and essential minerals we need. Green vegetables also contain a great deal of beta-carotenes and even some DHA fatty acid needed by the brain. Fruits and vegetables are important for maintaining the pH balance of the body. Chlorophyll contains a very high quantity of magnesium. Magnesium is to chlorophyll what iron is to hemoglobin in the blood—an oxygen carrier.

To asthmatics, people with osteoporosis, and also cancers, sunlight is medicine. Light from the sun acts on the cholesterol deposits on the skin and converts them to vitamin D. Vitamin D encourages bone making and the entrapment of calcium by the bones, which in children helps them grow. Vitamin D also stimulates calcium absorption in the intestinal tract. Calcium has a direct acid-neutralizing effect in the body and is effective in balancing the cell pH—an outcome that helps alleviate asthma complications.

If you drink adequate amounts of water every day, take the required amount of salt, and get plenty of exercise—preferably in the open air and under good light—your body will begin to adjust its own intake of proteins and carbohydrates, as well as its fat requirements to use for energy. Your need for proteins will increase. Your need for carbohydrates will decrease, and your fat-burning enzymes will consume more fat than is in the average diet. Contrary to the belief that cholesterol cannot be metabolized once it is deposited, it, too, will be cleared. The cholesterol deposits in the arteries may take longer to disappear than you might wish, but the body has all the chemical know-how to clear cholesterol plaques.

Cholesterol and Osteoporosis

Remember, cholesterol is vital to body physiology. We have to find out why the body manufactures more of it than usual. The following explanation is one of many I have found for this.

When there is a shortage of water in the body, less hydroelectric energy is manufactured to energize all

the dependent functions—much like low water flow
in the river that feeds an electricity-generating dam.
After a while, the dam will not hold enough water to
operate all the generators. In real-life situations, when
cheap energy from hydroelectric dams is insufficient,
power generators begin to burn oil or coal—dirty
fuel—to generate electricity.

In the body, the alternative source of energy is calcium deposits in the bone or inside the cells. The
energy trapped in the union of two calcium molecules
that are fused together is used instead. When two
calcium atoms bond together, one unit of ATP energy
is also trapped. The cells in the body have many
trapped bonded calcium atoms in different storage
sites that become broken up and their energy is used.
There comes a time when this process results in an
availability of too many loose calcium molecules—
similar to the ash of spent fuel. Fortunately, calcium
ash (so to speak) is easily recycled and, if energy is
available, calcium molecules bond together once
again and store energy for use—like charging a battery that is low.

Sunlight—energy—converts cholesterol in the
skin to vitamin D. Vitamin D is responsible for facilitating the reentrapment of calcium and its reentry
into the cells and the bones to be rebounded and
restored. Vitamin D sticks to its receptors on the cell
membrane; simultaneously, one unit of calcium
attaches itself to the exposed tail of the vitamin D that
is in the process of entering the cell through the cell
membrane. The union of calcium with vitamin D and
its membrane receptor acts as a sort of magnetic rod,

and whole chains of other essential elements and amino acids stick to the exposed calcium and are drawn into the cell.

In this way, the energy of sunlight, and its conversion of cholesterol to vitamin D, has a direct physiological impact on the feeding mechanism of the cells of the body. When calcium reenters the cell, it takes other essential elements with it. In this way, the cell receives raw materials for repair and energy metabolism. At the same time, the surplus energy that enters the cell is used to fuse together calcium molecules and once again store energy in the calcium bonds for future use.

Once you understand the logic behind the cascade of the chemical events in the body, you will realize the vital importance of cholesterol to cell metabolism and the health of the cells in the body. You should put the higher cholesterol levels of the body to full use by making more vitamin D from it and promoting better-functioning and fully energized and operational cells in your body. Use sunlight to your advantage to lower your cholesterol and promote formation of denser bones. Some of you might immediately react negatively to this statement and express your fear of melanoma. It is my thoughtful understanding that cancers in the body are produced by dehydration, inactivity, and poor choices of foods and beverages. For more than twenty years, I played three hours of tennis six days a week, in the heat of the early-afternoon sun in Tehran. I did not develop any form of cancer.

You cannot sit at a desk in an artificially lit office

and expect to have a normal cholesterol level and normal bone density in your body. And in this situation, you will probably have a health professional— one who does not understand the mechanisms and relationships of sunlight energy conversion—label this natural outcome of an incomplete chain of metabolic events a "disease"; a vital element, cholesterol, will also be labeled "bad."

Sunlight was first used successfully as medication when children with deformed bones (rickets) were exposed to it, which corrected the deformity. They called it heliotherapy. I interpret the gradual rise in cholesterol as we grow older through my scientific understanding of the many roles of cholesterol, and associate its increased production by the liver with the gradual decrease in bone density.

I think the rise in low-density cholesterol is a significant indicator of the onset of osteoporosis. To prevent osteoporosis, a gradual exposure to early-morning sunlight could be a natural way to increase calcium absorption into the body and the bones.

EXERCISE

The most important factor for survival, after air, water, salt, and food, is exercise. Exercise is more important to the health of the individual than sex, entertainment, or anything else that might be pleasurable. Here is why exercise is crucial for better health and a longer pain-free life:

- Exercise expands the vascular system in the muscle tissue and helps prevent hypertension.
- It opens the capillaries in the muscle tissue and, by lowering the resistance to blood flow in the arterial system, causes the blood pressure and blood sugar to drop to normal.
- Exercise builds up muscle mass—positive nitrogen balance—and prevents the muscles from being broken down as fuel.
- Exercise stimulates the activity of fat-burning enzymes for manufacturing constantly needed energy for muscle activity. When you train, you are in effect changing the source of energy for muscle activity. You convert the energy source from sugar that is in circulation to fat that is stored in the muscle itself, and elsewhere in the body.
- Exercise makes muscles burn as additional fuel some of the amino acids that would otherwise reach toxic levels in the body. In their greater-than-normal levels in the blood—usually reached in a sedentary body—certain branched-chain amino acids cause a drastic destruction and depletion of other vital amino acids. Some of these discarded essential amino acids are constantly needed by the brain to manufacture its neurotransmitters. Two of these essential amino acids are tryptophan and tyrosine. The brain uses tryptophan to make serotonin, melatonin, tryptamine, and indolamine, all of which are antidepressants and regulate sugar level and blood pressure. Tyrosine is used for the manufacture of adrenaline, noradrenaline, and dopamine—vital for the coordination of body physiology whenever it

has to take a physical action, such as fighting, running, playing sports, and so on. Tyrosine depletion is also a primary factor in Parkinson's disease.

- Unexercised muscle gets broken down. As a result of the excretion of muscle parts from the body, some of the reserves of zinc and vitamin B_6 also get lost. At a certain stage of this constant depletion of vitamin B_6 and zinc, certain mental disorders and neurological complications occur. In effect, this happens in autoimmune diseases, including lupus and muscular dystrophy.

- Exercise makes the muscles hold more water in reserve and prevents increased concentration of blood that would otherwise damage the lining of the blood vessel walls.

- Exercise lowers blood sugar in diabetics and decreases their need for insulin or tablet medications.

- Exercise compels the liver to manufacture sugar from the fat that it stores or that is circulating within the blood.

- Exercise causes an increase in the mobility of the joints in the body and creates an intermittent vacuum inside the joint cavities. The force of the vacuum causes suction of water into the cavity. Water in the joint cavity brings dissolved nutrients to the cells inside the cartilage. Increased water content of the cartilage also adds to its lubrication and smoother bone-on-bone gliding movements of the joint.

- Calf muscles act as secondary "hearts." By their contractions and relaxations when we are upright and moving, the leg muscles overcome the force of gravity. They pump into the venous system the blood that was sent to the legs. Because of the pressure breakers in the vein and one-directional valves, the blood in the leg veins is pushed upward against gravity by frequent contraction of the leg muscles. This is how the leg muscles act as a kind of heart for the venous system in the body. This is a value to exercise that not many people appreciate. Leg muscles also cause an equally effective flow within the lymphatic system and cause edema in the legs to disappear.

- Exercise strengthens the bones of the body and helps prevent osteoporosis.
- Exercise increases the production of all vital hormones, enhancing libido and heightening sexual performance.
- One hour of walking will cause the activation of fat-burning enzymes, which remain active for twelve hours. A morning and afternoon walk will keep these enzymes active around the clock and will clear cholesterol deposits in the arterial system, as well as fat from the fat stores in the body.
- Exercise will enhance the activity of the adrenaline-activated sympathetic nerve system. Adrenaline will also reduce the oversecretion of histamine and, as a result, will prevent asthma attacks and allergic reactions—providing the body is fully hydrated.
- Exercise will increase production of endorphins and enkephalins, the natural opiates of the body. They produce the same high that drug addicts try to achieve through their abusive intake.

What Are the Best Forms of Exercise?

Exercising the body for endurance is better than exercising it for speed or for building excess muscle. In selecting an exercise, you should consider its lifetime value. A long-distance runner will enjoy the exercise value of long-distance runs into old age. A sprinter will not sprint for exercise at a later phase of life.

The best exercise—one that you can benefit from even to a ripe old age, and without causing damage to your joints—is walking. Other exercises that will increase your endurance are swimming, golf, skiing, skating, climbing, tennis, squash, bicycling, tai chi, dancing, and aerobics. In selecting an exercise, evaluate its ability to keep the fat-burning enzymes active for longer durations. Outdoor forms of exercise are more beneficial for the body than indoor forms. The body becomes better connected to nature.

CONCLUSION:
Four Simple Steps to Vibrant Health

The four most vital steps to better health are balancing the *water* and *salt* content of the body; *exercising* the muscle mass of the body to enhance the efficiency of brain function; *avoiding beverages that dehydrate* and make the body more toxic; and eating a *balanced daily diet* of proteins and vegetables in a ratio of 20 percent protein and 80 percent vegetables, legumes, and fruits, with as little starch and sugar as possible. It is the high starch and sugar content of the diet that makes a person fat. *Higher protein and fat contents of the diet do not make you fat!*

If you stick to these recommendations, I am confident that you will seldom fall ill and will live a long and productive life.

I do hope you will share the information in this book with others who might need it.

INDEX